Physiotherapy for Burns
and Plastic Reconstruction of the Hand

For Mom and Dad

Physiotherapy
for burns and plastic reconstruction of the hand

Nicole Glassey MSc, Grad.Dip.Phys., MCSP

Clinical Specialist Physiotherapist, Nottingham City Hospital

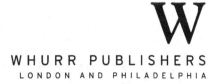

WHURR PUBLISHERS
LONDON AND PHILADELPHIA

© 2004 Whurr Publishers Ltd
First published 2004
by Whurr Publishers Ltd
19b Compton Terrace
London N1 2UN England and
325 Chestnut Street, Philadelphia PA 19106 USA

British Library Cataloguing in Publication Data

A catalogue record for this book
is available from the British Library.

ISBN 1 86156 386 8

Typeset by Adrian McLaughlin, a@microguides.net
Reprinted 2006

Contents

Preface

Newly qualified physiotherapists embark on at least two years of, on average, four-month clinical rotations throughout all the departments of their employing hospital. After the relief of qualifying, they become professionals in their own right and discover that learning is a life-long commitment for which they are responsible. Four months is a relatively short period of time for physiotherapists to become competent in each speciality and to enhance the knowledge they gained as students, in order to provide patients with the best possible care and treatment. This book is aimed at student physiotherapists, basic grade physiotherapists and Senior 2 physiotherapists who have no previous experience in burns and plastic surgery of the hand. The author's intention is to aid the continuation of learning by providing a greater depth of information than could have been studied at undergraduate level. The objective of the book is to provide a core text to be used during a burns and plastic surgery rotation, providing physiotherapists with the fundamental principles of therapy so that they can expand on this sound knowledge base with the experience they gain in clinical practice.

With the ever-increasing pressures of working within the NHS, and the recent greater emphasis on continuing professional development, senior members of staff find it difficult to allocate time from their working day to provide teaching and supervision for junior members of the team. This book attempts to ensure that junior members of staff understand the basic principles of treatment so that precious teaching time can be used in a more efficient and effective manner.

Acknowledgements

The author wishes to thank David Wilson FRCS, Alison Reeves, Eleanor Douglas and Cordelia Gaubert for their assistance in reviewing the text, Robert Duley and Matt Horobin for their assistance with photography and Jim McCarthy for his advice, support and encouragement.

Abbreviations

Anatomy

Abd	Abduction
Add	Adduction
ADM	Abductor digiti minimi
AED	Active extension deficit
AFD	Active flexion deficit
AP	Adductor pollicis
APB	Abductor pollicis brevis
APL	Abductor pollicis longus
CMC	Carpometacarpal
DES	Dynamic extension splint
DFS	Dynamic flexion splint
DIP	Distal interphalangeal
DRUJ	Distal radio-ulnar joint
ECRB	Extensor carpi radialis brevis
ECRL	Extensor carpi radialis longus
EDC	Extensor digitorum communis
EDM	Extensor digiti minimi
EI	Extensor indicis
EPB	Extensor pollicis brevis
EPL	Extensor pollicis longus
Ext	Extension
FCU	Flexor carpi ulnaris
FCR	Flexor carpi radialis
FDM	Flexor digiti minimi
FDP	Flexor digitorum profundus
FDS	Flexor digitorum superficialis
Flex	Flexion
FPB	Flexor pollicis brevis
FPL	Flexor pollicis longus

IF	Index finger
IP	Interphalangeal
LF	Little finger
MCP	Metacarpophalangeal
MF	Middle finger
NVB	Neurovascular bundle
ODM	Opponens digit minimi
OP	Opponens pollicis
PB	Palmaris brevis
PED	Passive extension deficit
PFD	Passive flexion deficit
PIP	Proximal interphalangeal
PL	Palmaris longus
POSI	Position of safe immobilization
PQ	Pronator quadratus
PT	Pronator teres
RCL	Radial collateral ligament
RF	Ring finger
Rot	Rotation
TAM	Total active motion
TPM	Total passive motion
UCL	Ulnar collateral ligament

Injury

CRPS	Complex regional pain syndrome
FTSL	Full thickness skin loss
PTSL	Partial thickness skin loss

Medical notes

Ax	Assessment
C/O	Complaining of
COD	Change of dressing
Cx	Conservative
D/C	Discharge
DNA	Did not attend
D/W	Discussed with
E/A	Emergency admission

ETOH   Alcohol
H/O   History of
ISQ   In status quo
Ix   Investigation
L   Left
Mx   Management
NAD   No abnormality detected
O/E   On examination
P   Pain
PCA   Patient-controlled analgesia
R   Right
R/A   Routine admission
ROS   Removal of sutures
Rx   Treatment
S/B   Seen by
UTA   Unable to attend
VAS   Visual analogue scale
↓   Decrease
Δ   Diagnosis
↑   Increase
∴   Therefore

Surgery

CTD   Carpal tunnel decompression
FTSG   Full thickness skin graft
MUA   Manipulation under anaesthetic
ORIF   Open reduction internal fixation
SSG   Split skin graft

Introduction

It is the aim of this book to present the principles of hand trauma and plastic reconstructive surgery in a clear, concise and essentially readable manner. It is assumed that, as final-year students or qualified physiotherapists, readers will have an adequate anatomical and biomechanical understanding of the body and, in particular, the hand. Although this may be elaborated upon in parts of the text it will not be dealt with individually. Obviously there are numerous injuries, conditions and treatment modalities that could be included in a book such as this but it is not the author's intention to produce an all-encompassing manual on the hand. This book is for student physiotherapists, basic grade physiotherapists and inexperienced Senior 2 physiotherapists who are beginning to develop their interest in hand trauma and who need a sound base of knowledge on which they can build further clinical experience and postgraduate study. Part 1 presents the principles of burns and plastic surgery, followed by an explanation of the role of the multidisciplinary team. Part 2 focuses on the role of the physiotherapist and includes the principles of hand therapy, assessment and treatment modalities.

This book differs to the majority of hand therapy books in that it does not list the injuries encountered most commonly and give prescriptive treatment regimes. The aim of the book is to instruct readers how to identify treatment priorities and, using the principles of therapy, how to select appropriate treatment modalities. Physiotherapists are encouraged to use a problem-solving method to develop treatment programmes and patients will receive treatment tailored to their needs. Treatment rationales are referenced with the available evidence, and aspects that lack evidence are highlighted with the intention of stimulating further investigation.

In order to clarify and reaffirm essential parts of the text, key points are made regularly throughout the book. These are fundamental to understanding the treatment of hand trauma, and are intended to be *aide mémoires* and easily accessed revision notes. At the end of the book, case studies are used to illustrate information. It is the author's experience that basic-grade physiotherapists relate to theory more easily if they see it demonstrated in clinical practice and it is with this in mind that cases and treatment programmes are discussed. Whilst studying these scenarios physiotherapists will soon discover that there are never simple hand injuries, usually any trauma to one structure affects several other tissues within the hand and upper limb, and physiotherapists are encouraged to develop a problem-solving approach to treating the whole patient not just the hand.

Part 1

Principles of burns and plastic surgery

Chapter 1

Tissue healing

Introduction

To manage any injury or condition effectively it is essential that physiotherapists understand the process of tissue healing. By knowing the rate at which the different tissues recover, physiotherapists can aid the process and be proactive in avoiding complications. Physiotherapists work with, and complement, the natural healing processes of the body, optimizing recovery. Because of the potentially catastrophic results of complications after hand trauma, physiotherapists should know when rest is required and when tissues need to be exercised, stretched or strengthened. Recognizing therapeutic effects on the healing process, and on the structures to which therapy is applied, is vital.

The body heals itself by the proliferation of fibrous tissue (scarring), which attempts to approximate normal anatomy. Tissue healing is a complex process and this chapter offers a brief overview of the salient events that occur during tissue healing in order to assist physiotherapists to recognize these stages clinically and to understand the possible effects that their treatment can have on the process.

Physiology of tissue healing

There are three stages of tissue healing:

- inflammation
- fibroplasia (proliferation)
- maturation (remodelling).

Inflammation

Inflammation is a complex response by the body tissues to any form of trauma, such as injury or infection. It is the clearing and preparatory stage that is necessary before wound healing can take place. During inflammation, micro-organisms and necrotic tissue are cleared from the injured area by the action of phagocytosing macrophages (Hardy, 1989).

Immediately after an injury, blood vessels constrict to prevent blood loss (Gibran and Heimbach, 2000). A period of vasodilation follows, to increase the circulation to the injured area and to supply all the necessary ingredients for healing. Undamaged blood vessels begin to sprout new buds and these grow into the injured area (Hardy, 1989). This angiogenesis is essential to supply nutrients to the healing tissues (Hardy, 1989). The release of chemical substances from the traumatized tissues attracts white blood cells to the area of injury, and the increased permeability of the capillaries allows these cells to pass into the tissue spaces. Exudate is formed, consisting of plasma that has leaked out of the capillaries and debris from dead white blood cells. Enzymes are released from the dead white blood cells and facilitate the breakdown of necrotic tissue. Fibroblasts begin to proliferate in preparation for collagen production.

Pus may be formed if there is a large presence of bacteria. The white blood cells and macrophages engulf the bacteria and wound debris but eventually die themselves. This combination of debris is pus. If a collection of pus is near to the surface of the skin, it will form an exit and drain out of the body; if the collection is deep within the tissues it will eventually be reabsorbed.

- *Duration*: 3–5 days.
- *Signs*: erythema, pain, heat, oedema.
- *Prolonged by*: debris, foreign matter; oedema; infection; ischaemia; poor nutrition; inappropriate dressings; rough handling or aggressive therapy; pre-existing conditions, such as diabetes; medications, such as steroids.
- *Treatment*: the aim of therapy intervention during this stage is to allow the inflammatory phase to subside as quickly as possible. Treatment should involve procedures that reduce pain and oedema, and prevent disruption of the delicate wound: minimal handling; positioning, e.g. splint; immobilization; elevation; wound care; nutrition.

Key point

An overzealous patient or physiotherapist can extend the inflammatory period, causing increased pain, stiffness and a reduction in function (Byron and Muntzer, 1986). The aim of inflammation is to clean the wound; once this is completed, healing can commence.

Fibroplasia (proliferation)

During fibroplasia, scar tissue begins to develop; this is the rebuilding phase (Hardy, 1989). Fibroblasts proliferate and endothelial budding continues to create new capillary growth. A framework of fibrin develops as fibroblasts produce a base gel and collagen. This collagen matrix and proliferation of the vasculature forms granulation tissue. Granulation tissue appears red, raised and moist; the newly formed vessels are often visible in the tissue (Pankhurst and Pochkhanawala, 2002). It is extremely delicate and will bleed easily. Collagen formation peaks at approximately 3 weeks and then levels off (Smith, 2002a). The synthesis of collagen becomes balanced with its degradation and tissue strength gradually increases (Smith, 2002a). Some of the fibroblasts become myofibroblasts and develop a contractile ability. This contraction (*see below*) draws the wound edges together and therefore decreases the size of the wound.

- *Duration*: begins at 3-5 days; lasts for 2-6 weeks.
- *Prolonged by*: infection; aggressive handling.
- *Treatment*: during early fibroplasia, positioning and immobilization prevent cell disruption (Smith, 1995a). However, once collagen development levels off and synthesis is balanced by degradation, gentle stress (such as splints and exercise) assists the development of collagen into a more favourable shape. Oedema will still be present and its resolution should continue to be a priority of therapy.

Contraction

The contractile properties of myofibroblasts cause the edges of a wound to be drawn together, reducing its size. In this way, the body protects itself by reducing the extent of damage that would otherwise allow fluid loss and provide an entry point for infection. In addition, the reduced size of the eventual scar aids cosmesis and tissue strength, as the scar tissue will never be as strong as the surrounding uninjured tissues (Smith, 2002a). The disadvantage to contraction of a wound is that if the injured area is over a joint, this contraction could limit the joint range of motion and eventually cause a joint contracture (*see* Chapter 6).

Maturation (remodelling)

The scar begins to change shape and strength. At the beginning of this process, the immature scar is bulky and comprises random collagen bundles. Remodelling orientates the collagen fibres along the lines of tension and they become more compact. The fibres do not actually move to orientate themselves. The change is accomplished by degradation of the random bundles and the synthesis of more uniform elongated bundles. This process can be assisted by the application of a gentle continuous stretch to the scar. Tensile strength gradually increases, and by 6 weeks, the scar has approximately 50% of the strength of normal tissue (Smith, 2002a; Pankhurst and Pochkhanawala, 2002), however, remodelling can continue for up to 2 years. Eventually the scar will become pale, pliable and soft.

- *Duration*: begins at 4–6 weeks; lasts for up to 2 years.
- *Signs*: early scar – red and raised; mature scar – flat, pale and pliable.
- *Treatment*: splinting; positioning; prevention of oedema; exercise, stretching, strengthening.

Key point

Stage of healing	Duration
Inflammation	3–5 days
Fibroplasia	2–6 weeks
Maturation	Up to 2 years

The three stages of tissue healing are not independent; they rely upon each other and overlap (*see* Figure 1.1 and Table 1.1.)

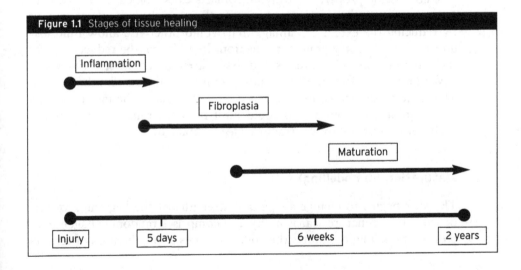

Figure 1.1 Stages of tissue healing

Table 1.1 The tissue healing process

Stage	Timescale	Process	Signs and symptoms
Inflammation	0–5 days	Blood vessels initially constrict then dilate to aid the influx of neutrophils and macrophages that will prevent infection and begin autolysis. Capillary permeability increases and exudate containing plasma, antibodies and white blood cells, leaks into the tissues	Erythema Oedema Heat Pain Reduced range of motion Reduced function
Destruction	2–5 days	Macrophages clear debris and initiate angiogenesis (Westaby, 1985)	As above
Fibroplasia (proliferation/ granulation)	5 days– 6 weeks	Fibroblasts synthesize collagen, which is laid down haphazardly. The increase in tensile strength parallels the increase in collagen production. Angiogenesis continues, leading to capillary budding and granulation tissue is formed	Moist, raised, red tissue in wound bed
Epithelialization	Primary closure: 2–48 hours Secondary intention: dependent on size of wound	Epithelial cells proliferate from the wound edges and any epithelial structures still present in the wound. The new cells migrate across the wound until complete coverage is achieved	Wound closure
Maturation	2 weeks– 2 years	Ongoing synthesis of collagen is balanced by degradation to allow organisation of the collagen fibres along the lines of stress, vascularity is reduced, and scar tissue strengthens	Scar flattens and becomes pale
Contraction	Wound: 4 to 5 days to 1 month Scar tissue: up to 2 years	Myofibroblasts provide the contractile force that initially reduces the size of the wound and eventually causes contraction of the resultant scar tissue	Wound reduces in size. Scar tissue becomes tight and, if over a joint, may result in a joint contracture if untreated

Specific tissue healing

Skin

The function of the hand is dependent on the versatility of the skin that covers it. For example, to facilitate motion within the hand the dorsal skin must be able to stretch over the flexed joints. In addition, to assist grip the palmar skin must contain sweat glands to create friction and nerve receptors to create sensory feedback.

A wound is a 'disruption of the anatomic or functional continuity of tissue' (Anthony, 1997).

Classification of wounds

- *tidy*: a clean laceration with minimal tissue damage, and uncontaminated.
- *untidy*: marked tissue damage, possibly involving some of the deeper structures, such as tendons, and often associated with contamination.
- *tissue loss*: significant tissue damage, involving deeper structures, could involve amputation.
- *infected*: gross contamination of a wound, exhibiting the classic signs and symptoms of infection – heat, erythema, pain, oedema and purulent exudate.

(For assessment of wounds, *see* Chapter 8.)

The skin has a remarkable ability to heal itself, although this is dependent upon the extent of tissue loss that is sustained. Cason (1981) reported that although large areas of tissue loss would eventually heal spontaneously, it could take months and even years, by which time the complications of an open wound may have seriously affected the patient's well-being and even endangered life. Therefore, surgical intervention may be necessary to speed up the rate of closure of a wound, and wound care products are used to facilitate the continuation of the natural biological healing process. The presence of necrotic tissue and debris within a wound will delay healing and increase the risk of bacterial infection. The body will attempt to clear this contamination and debris by autolysis (the natural ability of the body to degrade devitalized tissue), but if extensive, surgical debridement of a wound may be necessary (Pankhurst and Pochkhanawala, 2002).

Superficial skin loss involves the destruction of the epidermis only, which although very painful, will normally heal independently within 7–10 days. The epidermis is self-regenerating by mitosis. Epithelium from the edges of the wound and the remnants of epithelial structures such as hair follicles and sweat glands (Quinn et al., 1985) proliferate and gradually cover the wound until it is closed. Re-epithelialization occurs most effectively in a moist environment (Dziewulski, 1992). Pape (1993) stated that the loss of epithelial cellular contact caused by injury stimulates epithelialization (contact guidance) and that when the epithelial cells achieve coverage of the wound, epithelialization ceases (contact inhibition).

Partial skin loss involves the destruction of part of the dermis. Depending upon the extent of the loss of dermis, the injury is termed 'superficial partial thickness loss' or 'deep partial thickness loss (deep dermal loss)' (Dziewulski, 1992). In superficial partial thickness skin loss, epithelial structures (the hair follicles, sweat and sebaceous glands) are mostly intact and therefore aid re-epithelialization. However, in deep partial thickness skin loss these structures are virtually all destroyed except for the very deepest portions. Gradually the remaining dermal cells proliferate, eventually joining to cover the wound and epithelialize. Wound closure takes between 7 and 14 days after superficial partial thickness skin loss and slightly longer following deep partial thickness skin loss. The depth of the damage to the dermis is proportional to the extent of the scarring and therefore the potential for contractures. Hence, deep partial thickness wounds often require surgery to facilitate rapid wound closure, to prevent infection and to create a more acceptable scar. Partial thickness skin loss can become full thickness if the wound becomes infected or ischaemic.

Full thickness skin loss involves the destruction of the entire dermis and may even involve the subcutaneous tissues. None of the epidermal structures survive. This type of severe wound rarely heals without some form of surgical intervention, and if it does, healing takes many months and creates unacceptable scarring. Figure 1.2 shows the different depths of skin loss.

(For further classification of depths of skin loss, *see* Chapter 3.)

Cutaneous wound healing

Within 10 minutes of an injury, the damaged tissues release powerful enzymes that stimulate the healing process (Evans, 1980). The speed of natural wound healing cannot be influenced. The body's ability to heal itself can only be complemented by the use of appropriate dressings to prevent complications such as infection, and by the application of appropriate forces, such as exercise or splintage.

Dziewulski (1992) described the stages of healing of a cutaneous wound as:

- inflammation
- granulation
- epithelialization
- maturation.

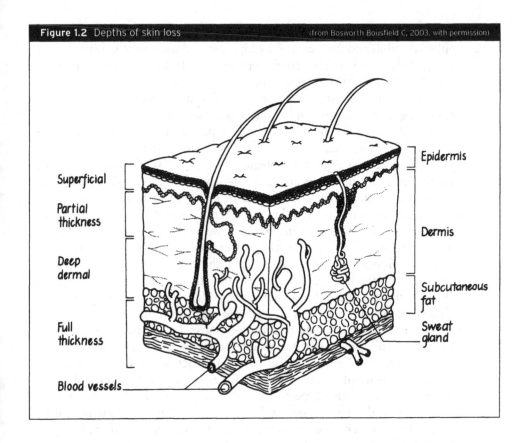

Figure 1.2 Depths of skin loss   (from Bosworth Bousfield C, 2003, with permission)

Superficial

Partial
thickness

Deep
dermal

Full
thickness

Blood vessels

Epidermis

Dermis

Subcutaneous
fat

Sweat
gland

Other authors give more extensive classifications of the stages of wound healing. For example, Pankhurst and Pochkhanawala (2002) note six stages of healing:

- inflammation
- destruction
- proliferation
- epithelialization
- maturation
- contraction.

(*See also* Table 1.1.)

Do not be confused by the variations in terminology in the literature, the process is the same! The ultimate aim of this process is the replacement of the lost dermis with scar tissue and the epidermis by re-epithelialization (Dziewulski, 1992). The easiest method of describing wound healing is within the three overlapping stages of any tissue healing:

- inflammation
- fibroplasia
- maturation.

Classification of wound closure

- *Secondary intention*: '... a wound is allowed to heal naturally without any surgical intervention. This is particularly beneficial when wound contraction is required to limit the size of scarring, for example fingertip injuries' (Connolly, 1974).
- *Primary closure*: immediate closure of a wound by suture or grafting.
- *Delayed primary closure*: a wound may be left open for as long as 5 days to allow resolution of oedema or infection before it is closed.

(*See* Chapter 4 for further details on classification of wound closure.)

Scarring

Scarring following an injury is inevitable. The extent of the scar depends on the depth and extent of the wound, but also on the individual. Azad et al. (2000) reported that the normal stages of scarring are:

- *Early*: fragile and prone to breakdown.
- *Mid*: red and raised.
- *Late*: thin and pale.

However, abnormal scarring is caused by an 'exaggerated response' to healing (Azad et al., 2000). The result of this exaggerated response is either hypertrophic or keloid scarring. The most common sites for excessive scarring are the ears, anterior neck, shoulders, chest and flexor surfaces of the extremities (Azad et al., 2000). This is thought to be caused by an increase in the tension across the scar, which increases fibroblast activity (Azad et al., 2000). Roehr et al. (1997) noted that both hypertrophic and keloid scarring is characterized by increased production of collagen tissue. This increase occurs because of increased synthesis associated with decreased degradation or a combination of the two. Table 1.2 describes different types of scars.

Table 1.2 Different types of scars

Hypertrophic	Keloid
Raised, red, itchy	Raised, red, itchy
Remain within area of injury	Extend beyond the boundaries of the injury
	More common in pigmented skin

It is difficult for clinicians to predict or prevent hypertrophic scarring (Gibran and Heimbach, 2000) but Gollup (1997) noted factors that affected scarring in individuals who suffered burns:

- *Age*: the young scar more severely.
- *Anatomical site of injury*: (see above).
- *Hair and skin colour*: the extremes of pigmentation are predisposed to scarring more extensively.
- *Infection*: delays healing and may result in a deeper injury (Ward and Saffle, 1995) therefore causing more extensive scarring.
- *Surgical intervention*: split skin grafts scar more readily than full thickness grafts or flaps (*see* Chapter 4).
- *Genetic factors*: some individuals are more susceptible to scarring; however, Roehr et al. (1997) noted that gender does not seem to influence scarring.

Blaha and Pondelicek (1997) also stated that the scarring that results from burns depends on:

- individual response to injury
- depth of injury
- site of injury
- early excision and grafting
- infection
- application of appropriate dressings
- use of pressure modalities (*see* Chapter 9)
- congenital predisposition to hypertrophy or keloid.

Bone

The bones of the hand are multiple and relatively small with numerous joints. Because of the potential for large forces being transmitted through these bones or joints through falls or the use of tools, for example, the bones of the hand and wrist are particularly susceptible to fractures.

Classification of fractures

Fractures can be classified according to their location, cause, stability, stage of healing and direction:

- *location*: diaphyseal, metaphyseal, articular
- *position*: neck, midshaft, base, intra-articular
- pathological or traumatic
- complete or incomplete

- open or closed
- stable or unstable
- displaced or undisplaced
- spiral, transverse, longitudinal, oblique
- simple or comminuted
- union or consolidation, non-union or mal-union.

Fractures do not strictly need to be immobile to heal. Within the hand, prolonged immobility can cause joint stiffness. As some movement at the fracture site will stimulate fracture healing, immobilization may be unnecessary. The purpose of splinting a fracture is not always to aid healing, but to reduce pain, maintain an optimum position and to permit early mobility and subsequent function (Apley and Soloman, 1993).

Fracture healing

As with any tissue, fracture healing can be described within the remit of the three stages of all tissue healing:

- *Inflammation*: bleeding into the marrow cavity and surrounding tissue forms a fracture haematoma. The tissues become oedematous, whereas the ischaemic bone ends die back slightly. Periosteum and endosteum proliferate to produce a bridge across the fracture site, and capillary proliferation provides increased vasculature to aid the provision of nutrients and absorption of the fracture haematoma.

- *Fibroplasia*: proliferation of periosteal and endosteal cells continues while osteoclasts begin the degradation of dead bone. Collagen synthesis forms a fibrous callus that bridges the bone fragments, limiting fracture site movement and forming a natural splint for the fracture (Apley and Soloman, 1993). Fracture union is achieved at approximately 4 weeks after injury (Apley and Soloman, 1993). Eventually, synthesis exceeds degradation and ossification provides stability.

- *Maturation*: gradually the bridge of solid bone is remodelled by re-absorption. It can take months or years to reshape the bone.

The duration of fracture healing is dependent upon the following:

- site of the fracture
- severity of the fracture
- amount of movement at the fracture site – some movement is beneficial as it will stimulate callus formation; however, too much movement could cause mal-union or non-union
- patient's age

- blood supply
- compliance with treatment.

On average, fractures of the bones in the hand and upper limb, require 4-6 weeks to unite.

Tendons

Tendon healing within the hand has been investigated and reported extensively, the plethora of research indicates its importance within the fields of hand surgery and physiotherapy. The function of the hand depends on the strength of the tendons and their ability to glide between the surrounding tissues.

Here, the healing of the flexor tendons of the hand is discussed, as this is most pertinent to hand physiotherapists. However, the theory of how tendons heal can be related to any tendinous structure within the body.

Tendon healing is a contradictory and controversial subject. The controversy over nutritional and healing pathways in tendons continues to be debated within the literature. There are three schools of thought concerning the process, relating to whether tendons have the potential to heal an injury themsleves or are reliant upon the influx of external adhesions:

- *intrinsic healing*: no extra-tendinous cellular participation
- *extrinsic healing*: extra-tendinous cellular participation only
- both intrinsic and extrinsic healing.

Most research into tendon healing is based on animal studies, therefore the extent to which intrinsic or extrinsic healing occurs in actual clinical practice is still unknown. Knowledge of the process of tendon healing will aid the application of appropriately timed therapeutic interventions.

Tendon nutrition

Healing flexor tendons receive nutrition from the digital vascular supply and the synovial fluid (Harris, 1998; Wagner and Strickland, 1999).

- *Digital vascular supply*: the extrinsic flexor tendons of the hand receive their blood supply from the vincula (small blood vessels that insert into the dorsal surface of the tendon), which are fed by branches of the digital arteries. The origins of the vincula are at the metacarpophalangeal and interphalangeal joint levels and their numbers vary from digit to digit, reducing with age (Amadio et al., 1995). Between the vincula there are avascular zones. Flexor tendon injuries that are associated with injury to the vincula system have a poorer prognosis than those in which the vincula remain uninjured (Amadio et al., 1995). The flexor tendons also derive a blood supply from the palmar vessels at the musculo-tendinous junction and from their distal bony insertion (Boscheinen-Morrin et al., 1992).

- *Synovial fluid*: Gelberman and Woo (1989) reported that although it was previously thought that flexor tendon nutrition in the hand was reliant upon the vincula system, there is evidence that synovial fluid has an important role in the healing process. Tendon injury frequently involves injury to the vincula system, resulting in increased avascular areas of tendon. However, if synovial nutrition is maintained, even avascular tendons may survive without restricting adhesions. Studies have indicated an important role for synovial fluid in tendon nutrition (Lundborg and Rank, 1980; Manske and Lesker, 1982).

- *Pulley system*: the role of the pulley system in the biomechanics of the flexor tendon system within the hand is well established. However, Amadio et al. (1995) reported a number of studies that noted the nutritional role of the pulleys. The provision of pressure on the volar aspect of the tendon surface by the pulleys (Amadio et al., 1995) creates lubrication and effectively pumps nutrients into the tendon.

Key point

Both vascular and synovial nutrition are necessary in tendon healing (Culp and Taras, 2002).

Tendon healing

Tendon consists of collagen bundles (70%) and elastic fibres surrounded by epitendon (Stewart Pettengill and van Strien, 2002). If a tendon is allowed to heal undisturbed, that is, without the application of any forces such as movement, it will heal but will adhere to all the surrounding structures and independent function will be lost.

Tendon healing is described by Wang (1998) and Stewart Pettengill and van Strien, (2002) within the three phases of tissue healing:

- *Inflammatory phase*: begins immediately after injury and lasts for approximately 3 days (Wang, 1998); alteration in vascular permeability (Stewart Pettengill and van Strien, 2002); leukocytes and macrophages converge on site of injury (Stewart Pettengill and van Strien, 2002) and phagocytose debris (Wang, 1998); proliferation of fibroblasts from outer edge of the tendon and surrounding tissue (Wang, 1998); fibrin clot forms (Wang, 1998); vascular proliferation within tendon (Stewart Pettengill and van Strien, 2002); collagen synthesis begins (Wang, 1998); the tensile strength of the tendon reduces in the first 3-5 days because of softening of the tendon ends (Stewart Pettengill and van Strien, 2002).

- *Fibroplastic phase*: commences 3-5 days after injury (Stewart Pettengill and van Strien, 2002); lasts for approximately 21 days (Wang, 1998); intrinsic angiogenesis from epitenon (Wang, 1998); synthesis of collagen in random patterns (Wang, 1998); collagen fibres bridge the repair at 10 days (Stewart Pettengill and van Strien, 2002).

- *Remodelling phase*: commences 3-4 weeks after injury (Wang, 1998); scar becomes more pliable; aided by gentle stress the collagen re-orientates (Wang, 1998); a passively mobilized tendon achieves 50% of normal strength at 12 weeks compared with an immobilized tendon achieving only 20% of same (Stewart Pettengill and van Strien, 2002); remodelling can last for 6 months to 1 year after injury (Stewart Pettengill and van Strien, 2002).

Extrinsic or intrinsic healing?

Research into tendon healing abounds and yet the exact mechanism of the process is still unknown. The contradictions within the literature concerning tendon nutrition have already been discussed, but there is also controversy over whether fibroblastic activity originates from within the tendon (intrinsic) or from the surrounding structures (extrinsic). Three mechanisms of tendon healing are presented below.

Intrinsic mechanism
Tendon healing occurs as a result of processes that originate from inside the tendon (Wang, 1998):

- proliferation occurs from the tenocytes and intratendinous vasculature (Wang, 1998)
- no adhesion formation (Wang, 1998)

Extrinsic mechanism
Tendon healing occurs as a result of processes that originate from outside the tendon (Wang, 1998):

- healing occurs via the formation of adhesions between the tendon and its surrounding structures (Stewart Pettengill and van Strien, 2002)
- fibroblasts originate from the surrounding tissues

- influenced by extratendinous vascular components (Wang, 1998)
- extrinsic healing – and hence adhesion formation – is exacerbated if there is excessive associated soft tissue trauma (Wang, 1998).

Combination of intrinsic and extrinsic mechanisms

Both intrinsic and extrinsic healing occurs simultaneously, complementing each other, to produce a strong tendon repair:

- the more intrinsic rather than extrinsic healing that takes place means fewer adhesions (Wagner and Strickland, 1999).

Variables that affect the outcome of a tendon repair

Stewart and van Strien (1995) reported a number of factors that influence tendon healing and the outcome of flexor tendon repairs in the hand:

- *age*: the number of vincula decreases with age, leading to larger areas of avascular tendon and reducing the potential for healing
- poor general health reduces the potential for healing
- smoking delays healing due to vasoconstriction
- caffeine delays healing due to vasoconstriction
- *scar formation*: individuals form scars differently with consequential differences in the formation of adhesions that will limit glide, pliability and mobility
- motivation and the patient's ability to comply with the post-operative exercise regime will determine the end result of a tendon repair
- *socio-economic factors*: family life and financial constraints may affect rehabilitation.

Effects of physiotherapy on tendon healing

The application of forces to a healing tendon risks rupture or repair site damage, but its aim is to produce the beneficial effects of increasing nutrition, tensile strength and to prevent interstructural adhesions. Traditionally, the immobilization of repaired structures has been advocated during the inflammatory phase of healing, followed by the application of controlled stresses during the fibroplastic phase, and an increase in the amount of force during the maturation phase. However, Gelberman et al. (1983) showed that early mobilization (even during the inflammatory phase) after a flexor tendon repair reduced adhesions, facilitated tendon glide and increased the tensile strength of the repair and the resultant range of motion achieved. Strickland (1989) also demonstrated that the application of appropriate stress influenced collagen synthesis and degradation. (For further detail on therapeutic intervention, *see* chapters 7 and 9.)

Nerve

Neural control of the hand provides both motor and sensory stimulus to the muscles, tendons, joints and skin in order to produce dexterity and strength. It is vital that physiotherapists treating patients with peripheral nerve injuries understand the nature of the injury and the healing mechanisms of the nervous system.

Common locations or causes of nerve injury are the following.

- *Digital nerves*: lacerations to digits.
- *Median nerve*: laceration at wrist level and compression within the carpal tunnel (carpal tunnel syndrome) or between the two heads of the pronator teres (pronator syndrome).
- *Ulnar nerve*: laceration at the wrist or elbow, and compression at the elbow (cubital tunnel) or the wrist (Guyon's canal).
- *Radial nerve*: nerve trauma accompanied by a fractured humerus and compression between the radial head and supinator (radial tunnel).

Different mechanisms of injury will result in a variety of levels of tissue damage that will alter the ultimate prognosis.

Classification of nerve injury by cause

- *Laceration*: caused by the traumatic application of, most commonly, a sharp instrument or bone fragment.
- *Crush or compression*: depending on the magnitude of force and the duration of exposure, this type of injury can result in any level of nerve damage (*see* classifications below). Not only is the nerve structure itself compressed, but its vascular supply will also be compromised and ischaemia will result.
- *Stretch*: nerves have the ability to glide between their surrounding structures during joint motion; however, they can be overstretched because of trauma or owing to their normal extensibility being limited by adhesions or entrapment.
- *Ischaemia*: as in any other anatomical structure, nerves are reliant upon the delivery of oxygen via the circulatory system. If this is occluded, permanent nerve damage may result.

(Smith, 2002b)

Classification of nerve injury by anatomical disruption

The two most common methods of classifying peripheral nerve injuries were described by Seddon (1943) and Sunderland (1968).

Seddon's classification

- *Neurapraxia*: anatomically the continuity of the nerve is maintained. The nerve is bruised and therefore its function is limited for a period of up to 6 weeks whilst it recovers.
- *Axonotmesis*: the epineurium is intact but the axons within are disrupted.
- *Neurotmesis*: both the axons and the epineurium are disrupted. For recovery to be effective, surgical repair of the nerve is necessary.

Sunderland's classification

1. Identical to Seddon's neuropraxic level of injury.
2. Identical to Seddon's axonotmetric level of injury.
3. Nerve fibres and endoneurium are disrupted.
4. Nerve fibres, endoneurium and perineurium are disrupted.
5. Complete disruption of all the nerve structures.

Key point

Classification	Damaged structures
Neuropraxia	Bruised but anatomically intact
Axonotmesis	Axonal disruption
Neurotmesis	Axonal and epineural disruption

Peripheral nerve healing

Nerve recovery occurs by a period of degeneration followed by a period of regeneration. This process takes place for both axonotmetric and neurotmetric injuries. After damage to the peripheral nerve, degeneration occurs in the proximal portion to the level of the first node of Ranvier (Irwin, 1999). The distal portion of the axon degenerates, but the remaining Schwann cell sheath directs the regenerating axonal fibres from the proximal portion of the nerve (Smith, 1995b). If the epineurium is disrupted it will need to be repaired surgically to facilitate optimal regeneration. If surgical repair has been necessary, the nerve should be protected from movement for approximately 3 weeks (Boscheinen-Morrin and Conolly, 2001).

Regeneration commences almost immediately after injury (Irwin, 1999). The tip of the axon buds and sends out projections that then proceed distally towards the target organ (Irwin, 1999). As the nerve grows distally, the Schwann cells also progress distally and are believed to help guide the axon towards their target (Irwin, 1999). The regenerating nerve grows at a rate of 1–3 mm a day (Irwin, 1999). The site of injury determines the rate of recovery of motor and sensory function. This must be explained to patients so that they are aware of the length of time necessary before they can expect any recovery. Even once the regenerating nerve reaches its target there will be a period of maturation before reinnervation is complete.

Key point

Approximate healing times according to site of injury:

digital nerve injuries to recover: 6 months
wrist level: 12–18 months
higher lesions: 2 years plus

Factors affecting nerve recovery

- scar tissue can block a regenerating nerve
- delayed surgical repair causes increased scarring in the distal portion of the nerve
- *age*: young patients tend to have a better prognosis
- *level of injury*: proximal injuries have a poorer prognosis because of the greater distance of regeneration to the target organ
- *tension of repair*: reduces blood flow and causes gapping between the nerve ends, leading to ischaemia and reduced healing (Irwin, 1999)
- cause of injury
- surgical technique.

References

Amadio PC, Jaeger SH, Hunter JM (1995) Nutritional aspects of tendon healing. In: JM Hunter, EJ Mackin, AD Callahan Rehabilitation of the Hand: Surgery and Therapy. St Louis, MI: Mosby.

Anthony MS (1997) Wound care. In: GL Clark, EF Shaw Wilgis, B Aiello, D Eckhaus, L Valdata L Eddington Hand Rehabilitation. A Practical Guide (second edition). London: Churchill Livingstone.

Apley AG, Soloman L (1993) Apley's System of Orthopaedics and Fractures. Oxford: Butterworth-Heinemann.

Azad SM, Gerrish J, Dziewulski P (2000) Hypertrophic scars and keloids: an overview of the aetiology and management. British Journal of Hand Therapy 5: 16-20.

Blaha J, Pondelicek I (1997) Prevention and therapy of postburn scars. Acta Chirurgiae Plasticae 39: 17-21.

Boscheinen-Morrin J, Davey V, Connolly WB (1992) The Hand: Fundamentals of Therapy (second edition). Oxford: Butterworth-Heinemann.

Boscheinen-Morrin J, Connolly WB (2001) The Hand: Fundamentals of Therapy (third edition). Oxford: Butterworth-Heinemann.

Byron PM, Muntzer EM (1986) Therapists' management of the mutilated hand. Hand Clinics 2: 69-79.

Cason JS (1981) Treatment of Burns. London Chapman & Hall.

Connolly WB (1974) Spontaneously healing and wound contraction of soft tissue wounds of the hand. Hand 6: 26-32.

Culp RW, Taras JS (2002) Primary care of flexor tendon injuries. In: EJ Mackin, AD Callahan, TM Skirven, LH Schneider, AL Osterman Rehabilitation of the Hand and Upper Extremity (fifth edition). St Louis, MI: Mosby.

Dziewulski P (1992) Burn wound healing: James Ellsworth Laing memorial essay for 1991. Burns 18: 466-74.

Evans P (1980) The healing process at cellular level: a review. Physiotherapy 66: 256-9.

Gelberman RH, Woo SL-Y (1989) The physiological basis for application of controlled stress in the rehabilitation of flexor tendon injuries. Journal of Hand Therapy, Apr-Jun: 66-70.

Gelberman RH, Vandberg JS, Lundborg GN et al. (1983) Flexor tendon healing and restoration of the gliding surface. An ultrastructural study in dogs. Journal of Bone and Joint Surgery 65A: 70-80.

Gibran NS, Heimbach DM (2000) Current status of burn wound pathophysiology. Clinics in Plastic Surgery 27: 11-22.

Gollup R (1997) Burns aftercare and scar management. In: C Bosworth Burns Trauma: Management and Nursing Care. London: Baillière Tindall.

Hardy MA (1989) The biology of scar formation. Physical Therapy 69: 1014-24.

Harris S (1998) Influences on flexor tendon rehabilitation. British Journal of Hand Therapy 3: 10-11.

Irwin MS (1999) Nerve repair and regeneration. British Journal of Hand Therapy 4: 8-12.

Lundborg G, Rank F (1980) Experimental studies on cellular mechanisms involved in healing of animal and human flexor tendon in synovial environment. Hand 12: 3-11.

Manske PR, Lesker PA (1982) Nutrient pathways of flexor tendons in primates. Journal of Hand Surgery 7: 436-44.

Pankhurst S, Pochkhanawala T, (2002) Wound care. In: C Bosworth Bousfield Burns Trauma: Management and Nursing Care (second edition). London: Whurr Publishers.

Pape SA (1993) The management of scars. Journal of Wound Care 2(6): 354-60.

Quinn KJ, Courtney JM, Evans JH, Gaylor JDS (1985) Principles of burn dressing. Biomaterials 6: 369-77.

Roehr SP, Khan U, Healy CMJ (1997) Scars and scar revision. British Journal of Hand Therapy 2: 4-8.

Seddon HJ (1943) Three types of nerve injury. Brain 66: 237.

Smith KL (1995a) Wound care for the hand patient. In: JM Hunter, EJ Mackin, AD Callahan Rehabilitation of the Hand: Surgery and Therapy. St Louis, MI: Mosby.

Smith KL (1995b) Nerve response to injury and repair. In: JM Hunter, EJ Mackin, AD Callahan Rehabilitation of the Hand: Surgery and Therapy. St Louis, MI: Mosby.

Smith KL (2002a) Wound care for the hand patient. In: EJ Mackin, AD Callahan, TM Skirven, LH Schneider, AL Osterman Rehabilitation of the Hand and Upper Extremity (fifth edition). St Louis, MI: Mosby.

Smith KL (2002b) Nerve response to injury and repair. In: EJ Mackin, AD Callahan, TM Skirven, LH Schneider, AL Osterman Rehabilitation of the Hand and Upper Extremity (fifth edition). St Louis, MI: Mosby.

Stewart KM, van Strien G (1995) Post-operative management of flexor tendon injuries. In: JM Hunter, EJ Mackin, AD Callahan Rehabilitation of the Hand: Surgery and Therapy. St Louis, MI: Mosby.

Stewart Pettengil KM, van Strien G (2002) Post-operative management of flexor tendon injuries. In: EJ Mackin, AD Callahan, TM Skirven, LH Schneider, AL Osterman Rehabilitation of the Hand and Upper Extremity (fifth edition). St Louis, MI: Mosby.

Strickland JW (1989) Biologic rationale, clinical application, and results of early motion following flexor tendon repair. Journal of Hand Therapy Apr-Jun: 71-83.

Sunderland S (1968) Nerves and nerve injuries. Edinburgh: E&S Livingstone.

Wagner WF, Strickland JW (1999) Flexor tendon injuries. In: J Weinzweig Plastic Surgery Secrets. Philadelphia, PA: Hanley & Belfus, chapter 93.

Wang ED (1998) Tendon repair. Journal of Hand Therapy Apr-Jun: 105-10.

Ward RS, Saffle JR (1995) Topical agents in burn and wound care. Physical Therapy 75: 526-38.

Westaby S (1985) Wound Care. London: Heineman.

Chapter 2

Hand trauma

Introduction

Trauma to the hand presents a challenge to surgeons, physiotherapists and patients. The hand is one of the most common areas of the body to sustain an injury because its use as a functional tool brings it into contact with potentially hazardous activities. In addition, hands are used to protect the rest of the body from injury or assault.

Methods of injury

Accident

This is by far the most common method of injury to the hand. Harvey Kemble and Lamb (1984) reported that 75% of burn injuries resulted from domestic accidents. Despite developments in health and safety legislation, safety devices being included in the manufacture of machinery and household goods, greater awareness of potential hazards and education on first aid, accidents continue to happen.

Assault

Hand injuries resulting from assault usually occur because the hand is used to protect the body, that is, defence injuries. Burn injuries are most commonly perpetrated among vulnerable groups of people, such as children or the elderly. These assaults are termed non-accidental injuries (NAI). The relevant authorities should be notified and all members of the multidisciplinary team should be advised if NAIs are suspected.

Deliberate self-harm

Patients who have deliberately injured themselves require a huge amount of support during their recovery and rehabilitation. A lot of support will be provided by the psychiatric department, but all members of the multidisciplinary team need to be involved in their recovery.

Prevention

Most hand injuries are preventable. Health and safety guidelines have reduced the number of injuries in the home and workplace, but further work is needed in this area. Simple measures, such as the installation of smoke detectors and the use of flame-retardant materials in furnishings and clothing, would reduce the number of burn injuries. The correct use of machinery and the wearing of protective clothing would reduce the number of work-related injuries.

Epidemiology

Young men seem to be more susceptible to hand injuries – probably because of the nature of their work and leisure activities (such as DIY and sports). People at the extremes of age are also more vulnerable to burn injuries. Children are commonly scalded by pulling hot drinks over themselves or climbing into hot baths. These accidents occur as children become more mobile but are still unaware of potential hazards. The elderly are more susceptible to injury owing to their frailty and loss of mobility. Other groups that are vulnerable to burn injuries are those with epilepsy, drug abusers, diabetic people and the mentally ill. MacArthur and Moore (1975) found that the aetiology of burn injuries is linked to individuals' physical, psychological and social well-being.

Hand trauma

There are numerous types of hand trauma; however, for the purposes of this chapter the most commonly encountered types of injury will be discussed:

- lacerations

- crushing
- degloving
- burns.

Lastly, as infection is a common complication of hand trauma (no matter what the cause), this is also discussed.

Lacerations

There is not usually any skin loss after a simple laceration from a sharp implement. However, depending upon the direction of the cutting force, there may be a raised part of the cutaneous tissue, termed a 'flap'. The extent of the trauma depends on the location of the injury and its depth. Injuries resulting from sharp implements are normally tidy (*see* classification of wounds, Chapter 1, and assessment of wounds, Chapter 8) and, once deeper structures have been repaired, these wounds are normally suitable for direct closure (McGregor and McGregor, 2000).

Crush injuries

The extent of trauma after a crush injury to the hand depends on the level and duration of force applied to the tissues. The immediate concern is the state of perfusion to the hand. Severe crush injuries result in extensive soft tissue damage and possibly bony injuries as well. Damage to the vasculature results in ischaemia of the tissues, and necrosis. Crush injuries are also marked by extensive oedema. The combination of lost tissue caused by ischaemia and extensive fibrosis because of oedema often leads to a poor result despite appropriate rehabilitation.

Degloving injuries

McGregor and McGregor (2000) define 'degloving' as trauma confined to the skin and fascia, but which is characterized by disruption to the vasculature of the tissue. It is unlikely that the degloved tissue can be salvaged and it often needs debridement followed by reconstructive surgery (*see* Chapter 4). Commonly, the skin from a single digit will be degloved if a ring is caught and dragged off. Often, amputation of the digit is the only option after such an injury, but if the vessels remain intact, microvascular surgery may save it (McGregor and McGregor, 2000).

Burn injuries

Types of burn injuries

Scald: The injury is sustained by the contact of a heated liquid with the skin. More often than not the liquid involved is water, but it can be any hot liquid, such as hot oil. Liquids have different boiling temperatures and are used at different heats. For example, a hot oil such as cooking oil will reach a higher temperature than boiling water and can therefore cause a deeper injury. Also, one of the most common scald injuries is caused by spilling hot drinks. The extent of damage depends upon whether the drink has been spilt immediately after it was made or whether it had been standing for a while, and had a cold fluid such as milk added to it, thus allowing some degree of cooling. It is important that a full and accurate history of an injury is taken, so that the extent and possible depth of a burn can be assessed.

Another common scald injury occurs when people get into a bath that is too hot. This usually happens to children, who climb into the bath before their parents have tested the temperature of the water. The extent of injury depends on the proportion of the body surface area that is immersed in the water, but is also affected by the temperature of the hot water supply to the bath. An easy way to avoid this situation is never to run a bath with hot water only, the cold water should always be run simultaneously, or the water heating system should be adjusted to ensure that the water temperature is not too hot. It is not only the young who can sustain scalds in the bath: once in the bath, elderly people may be unable to turn off the hot water or may be unable to get out of the bath without assistance.

Flame: the simplest mode of flame injury is a flash burn, which as it suggests is a momentary ignition of a fuel – most commonly petrol – and its vapour, causing a ball of flames that is quickly extinguished because of a lack of fuel, which can cause injury to anyone in the vicinity. Harvey Kemble and Lamb (1984) reported that even with a momentary exposure of more than 60°C, irreversible skin damage could occur. There is also a risk that the flash could ignite other materials in the area, such as clothing, causing more extensive tissue damage.

To be maintained a fire requires fuel and oxygen. Unfortunately, both are found in abundance in the home, in the workplace and among modes of transport, leading to devastating fires that spread quickly and reach tremendous temperatures. Despite legislation to improve fire safety, and the development of smoke and fire alarms, accidents still happen and the consequences of flame injuries to patients are devastating.

Contact: normally, if a part of the body encounters something that is hot, it causes pain, and the body part is removed immediately, thus preventing tissue damage. However, if for some reason the victim is unable to break the contact or is unable to feel the painful sensation, tissue damage will occur. The extent of tissue damage depends on the temperature of the surface and duration of the contact with it. Victims may not withdraw from a hot surface because:

- They have an area of anaesthetic skin caused by previous neurological damage, they cannot feel pain and do not realize that they are touching something hot, for example a person with a previous injury to the ulnar nerve will not be able to detect heat if they rest the ulnar border of the hand on a hot surface.

- They may be physically unable to move away from the hot surface, for example an elderly or infirm person may fall against a radiator and be unable to get up without help.

- They may have a reduced level of consciousness, or be unconscious, and unaware of the heat until they recover, for example someone who suffers with epilepsy may have a fit and fall onto a heated surface.

Radiation: the most common form of radiation burn is sunburn – either directly from the sun or from sunbeds (Cook, 2002). Another possible route of injury from radiation is radiotherapy.

Chemical: chemical burns occur most commonly in the workplace, where a variety of substances are used, in particular in the manufacturing and cleaning industries. Chemicals are also found in the home in cleaning, gardening and decorating products. If chemicals are used in the workplace, health and safety regulations ensure that staff are taught appropriate first aid. However, in the home, although potentially hazardous products have first aid instructions written on the packaging, these are often not read until after the event.

The extent and depth of injury caused by the contact of a chemical with the tissues depends on the amount of the chemical that comes into contact with the skin, the type of chemical, and its effects, and the timing of application of appropriate first aid. Most chemicals can be washed off the skin with water, but some substances react with water and cause deeper damage (Salisbury and Dingeldein, 1993). If these types of chemicals are being used the appropriate antidotes should be readily available. Examples of chemical burns include acids, alkali, ammonia, tar, cement burns and extravenous injection injuries from cytotoxic drugs.

Electrical: Chung et al. (1996) stated that 4% of admissions to burns units were caused by electrical injuries, and that these injuries most commonly affected the hands and upper limbs. Electrical injuries can be caused by low-voltage electrical appliances such as those found in the home, or by high-voltage currents, for example from high-tension overhead or underground cables.

The immediate concern after someone sustains a high-voltage electrical injury is the effect upon the cardiovascular system. By its nature, electricity attempts to earth itself. Therefore, on entry to the body, the electric current travels through the tissues that provide the least electrical resistance, that is, the blood vessels, muscle (Harvey Kemble and Lamb, 1984) and nerves, towards the earth. For this reason, examination of a patient who has sustained an electrical injury will normally reveal a visible entry wound and an exit wound. However, these obvious cutaneous wounds do not reveal the true extent of the injury to the deeper structures. As the electric current passes through the body it can destroy the tissues that aid its progress and the organs it passes through, most notably the heart. The heart is regulated by electrical impulses and its rhythm can be seriously disturbed or stopped by the passage of an electric current. All victims of an electrical injury should be monitored for cardiac arrhythmias.

Once the patient is cardiovascularly stable, the extent of the internal damage to the tissues needs to be assessed, as the electrical current may have destroyed the nerves and the highly vascular structures, for example musculature, without revealing a huge amount of skin damage.

Harvey-Kemble and Lamb (1987) describe the processes by which the tissues are damaged by electrical injury:

- direct heat damage by the passage of the current through the tissues
- ischaemic necrosis owing to damage to the vasculature
- electrical conductivity interference, for example to the heart or nerves
- tetanic contraction of the muscles – could be so severe that rupture or avulsion injury occurs
- ignition of clothing, leading to cutaneous flame burns
- propulsion of the body, leading to further bony or soft tissue injury.

Friction: friction burns are caused by the skin being dragged along a surface. These occur most commonly as a result of road traffic accidents. The extent and depth of the injury depends on the distance the victim was dragged and the texture of the surface where the accident occurred.

Cold: although cold trauma, or frostbite, is not common in the UK, it does occur and requires specialist treatment. The extent of tissue damage depends on the length of time the sufferer was exposed to the cold, and at what temperatures. Often, the only option is amputation of the affected parts. However, surgeons involved in the treatment of patients with frostbite will not rush into performing any operative procedure as it can take months for areas of tissue necrosis to demarcate between dead and healthy tissue, thus permitting assessment and a decision to be made about the required levels of amputation.

Modes of burn injury include scald, flame, contact, radiation, chemical, electrical, friction and cold.

First aid for burn injuries

The appropriate method of first aid after a burn trauma depends on the mode of injury. Applying appropriate first aid for an adequate length of time can make the difference between life and death. However, appropriate first aid can also make a difference concerning:

* superficial or deep burns
* needing conservative rather than surgical intervention
* the extent of scarring
* the psychological effect on the patient.

The aim of 'first' aid is to stop the burning process, to cool the burn and then to cover the wound.

Scald: the saturated clothing should be removed and the area of injury immersed under cool, running water for at least 10 minutes (Harvey Kemble and Lamb, 1984; Lawrence, 1996, Wilson, 2002). However, Sawada et al. (1997) demonstrated that excessive cooling of scald injuries, such as the immediate application of an ice cube to the wound, caused more severe tissue damage than if first aid had not been instituted.

Flame: lying the victim down and smothering the flames with either a blanket or by rolling them on the floor should extinguish the fire. The area of injury should then be immersed under cool, running water for at least 10 minutes. Clothing may stick to wounds and its removal could exacerbate tissue trauma and be very painful.

Contact: contact with a heat source should be broken and the injured area immersed in cool, running water for at least 10 minutes.

Chemical: for most chemicals, applying water to the affected area is indicated. However, some chemicals (for example, those containing metallic sodium or potassium) ignite when in contact with water (Harvey Kemble and Lamb, 1984), therefore an antidote is required. It is important to establish the exact chemical that caused the trauma.

Electrical: the electrical current must be broken, but this must be done without endangering the rescuer. Once the contact has been broken, it is vital that the victim's cardiovascular state is assessed and treated. For this to be done effectively the victim should be transferred to the nearest hospital with a casualty department.

Cold: the sufferer should be wrapped in warm garments. The extremities can be re-warmed rapidly in water at a temperature of 38°C (Harvey Kemble and Lamb, 1987). The re-warming process will be painful so analgesia or sedation may be necessary.

Once the appropriate first aid has been administered to stop the burning process and cool the injury, wounds should be covered with clingfilm (Wilson, 2002). The advantages of clingfilm are that the wound can be viewed through it, it prevents air reaching the nerve endings in the wound and therefore aids analgesia, it is non-adherent and easily removed. The victim should then be transferred to the nearest accident and emergency department.

Severity of burn injury

The severity of the burn sustained depends on the following:

- depth of burn
- extent of burn
- age of victim; those aged under 2 and over 60 have a higher mortality rate because their skin is thin, their immune response is poor and they are prone to infection; their protein stores may be minimal and are depleted quickly
- past medical history, pre-existing medical conditions (such as malnutrition, anaemia or diabetes) may affect the ability of the body to heal
- associated injuries, for example if victims have had to escape from a building they may have lacerations and fractures, the tetanic muscle contraction of electrical injuries can also cause fractures, an electric current can throw victims a fair distance leading to further injuries, and victims may have been involved in a road traffic accident followed by a fire
- location of burn; areas such as the eyes, face, hands, feet and perineum require specialized care

(Trofino, 1991).

Depth of burn injury

The depth of the burn sustained depends on the following:

- the burning agent, for example in chemical burns, the more destructive the chemical the deeper the burn
- the temperature of the agent: hot fat is used at higher temperatures than hot water

- the duration of exposure: synthetic materials retain heat for longer than natural fibres
- the conductivity of the tissue
- the thickness of the dermal tissue involved: dermal tissue is thicker on the palms of the hands and the soles of the feet.

(Trofino, 1991).

(For classification of the depth of skin loss and wounds, *see* chapters 1 and 3; for classification of the extent of injury, *see* Chapter 3; for the assessment of wounds, *see* Chapter 8.)

Infection

We have already seen that the hand is susceptible to constant exposure to risks of injury and this also means potential infections. Once the skin is broken, organisms can easily gain access to the body. These organisms may already reside on the skin or may be introduced as contaminants (Linscheid and Dobyns, 1975). Contaminating organisms can be bacterial, viral or fungal (Byrne, 1986). The most common pathogens that cause wound infection are *Staphylococcus aureus* (Weinzweig and Gonzalez, 1999) and Streptococcus (Nathan and Taras, 1995). Neglected or inadequately treated minor injuries can develop into serious infections that will result in extensive tissue destruction, scarring and, therefore, loss of hand motion and function. To establish the origin of an infection it is important to know the posture of the hand at the time of injury. For example, if the hand was clenched in a fist at the time of trauma, as in a punch injury, the site of structural damage or infection may not correspond to the external cutaneous wound. This is because the loose dorsal skin stretches distally during finger flexion but returns proximally on relaxation of the digits.

Key point

Signs of infection include erythema, heat, pain, pus, oedema and odour.

Treatment of infections

After recognizing an infection, rapid, appropriate treatment is essential. Current recommended treatments include the administration of either topical or systemic antibiotics, surgical drainage or debridement, irrigation and rehabilitation.

Common hand infections

Paronychia: infection of the nail fold, presenting with pain and swelling. If left untreated the accumulation of pus can lift the nail. Treatment is by drainage.

Subcutaneous abscess: can occur anywhere in the hand but the most common is termed a 'felon'. This is a subcutaneous abscess in the area of the distal phalanx. The pulp becomes extremely painful, red and swollen, and can result in extensive tissue necrosis. Surgical drainage is usually necessary.

Deep space infections: the fascial spaces of the hand, for example the radial and ulnar bursae, Parona's space, thenar space, etc., are at risk of infection, and pus can accumulate there. The connections between the deep spaces of the hand can lead to extension of the infection, for example an infection in the ulnar bursa can spread to the radial bursa and Parona's space – leading to a horseshoe infection.

Flexor sheath infection: infection in the flexor sheath will cause tendon adhesions and possibly tendon necrosis or rupture if treated inadequately. Kanavel (1925) described the four signs of flexor sheath tenosynovitis:

- pain affecting the sheath
- pain on passive digit extension
- digit held in flexed position
- oedema of digit.

The outcome following a flexor sheath infection depends on early recognition and treatment. The recommended management of an acute flexor sheath infection is surgical exploration, drainage and irrigation, followed by a period of post-operative irrigation and then vigorous rehabilitation (Neviaser, 1993; Jebson, 1998).

Complications of hand infections include the following:

- extension of infection throughout the hand
- soft tissue adhesion
- scarring
- reduced sensation
- tissue necrosis
- osteomyelitis.

References

Byrne JJ (1986) Hand infections – the academic surgeon's perspective – 2: a rundown of various causes. Postgraduate Medicine 80: 112–19.

Chung KC, Robson MC, Smith DJ (1996) Management of thermal, electrical, radiation and chemical injuries. In: CA Peimer Surgery of the Hand and Upper Extremity. London: McGraw-Hill.

Cook D (2002) Classification of burn trauma. In: C Bosworth Bousfield Burns Trauma: Management and Nursing Care (second edition). London: Whurr Publishers.

Harvey Kemble JV, Lamb BE (1984) Plastic Surgical and Burns Nursing. London: Baillière Tindall.

Harvey Kemble JV, Lamb BE (1987) Practical Burns Management. London: Hodder & Stoughton.

Jebson PJ (1998) Deep subfascial space infections. Hand Clinics 14: 557–66.

Kanavel AB (1925) Infections of the Hand: a Guide to the Surgical Treatment of Acute and Chronic Suppurative Processes in the Fingers (fifth edition). London: Baillière Tindall & Cox.

Lawrence JC (1996) First aid measures for treatment of burns and scalds. Journal of Wound Care 5: 319–22.

Linscheid RL, Dobyns JH (1975) Common and uncommon infections of the hand. Orthopedic Clinics of North America 6: 1063–1104.

MacArthur JD, Moore FD (1975) Epidemiology of burns, the burn prone patient. JAMA 231: 259–63.

McGregor AD, McGregor IA (2000) Fundamental Techniques of Plastic Surgery and their Surgical Applications (tenth edition). Edinburgh: Churchill Livingstone.

Nathan R, Taras JS (1995) Common infections of the hand. In: JM Hunter, EJ Mackin, AD Callahan Rehabilitation of the Hand: Surgery and Therapy. London: Mosby.

Neviaser RJ (1993) Infections. In: DP Green Operative Hand Surgery (third edition). London: Churchill Livingstone.

Salisbury RE, Dingeldein GP (1993) The burned hand and upper extremity. In: DP Green Operative Hand Surgery. London: Churchill Livingstone.

Sawada Y, Urushidate S, Yotsuyanagi T, Ishita K (1997) Is prolonged and excessive cooling of a scalded wound effective? Burns 23: 55–8.

Trofino RB (1991) Nursing Care of the Burn-injured Patient. Philadelphia, PA: FA Davies.

Weinzweig N, Gonzalez MH (1999) Infections of the hand. In: J Weinzweig Plastic Surgery Secrets. Philadelphia, PA: Hanley & Belfus.

Wilson D (2002) Management in the first 48 hours. In: C Bosworth Bousfield Burns Trauma: Management and Nursing Care (second edition). London: Whurr Publishers.

Chapter 3

Pathophysiology and assessment of burns

Pathophysiology of burns

The systemic effects that result from a burn injury cause catastrophic damage to the body. However, it is beyond the scope of this text to review each system individually but those that are pertinent to the hand will be discussed.

Further reading

- Bosworth Bousfield C (2002) Burns Trauma: Management and Nursing Care (second edition). London: Whurr Publishers.
- Settle JAD (1996) Principles and Practice of Burns Management. London: Churchill Livingstone.

Burn site pathophysiological changes

At the site of the injury, the wound is initially sterile because of the extreme temperature that has caused the trauma. However, once exposed to the environment the wound can easily become infected by contamination and colonization from micro-organisms (Staphylococcus, Pseudomonas, Streptococcus), as the protection normally afforded by the skin has been lost.

Immediately after a burn injury, the normal inflammatory process that initiates healing commences (*see* Chapter 1). In an attempt to dissipate the heat, the blood vessels vasodilate (Settle, 1996). Oedema occurs within the tissues because of the increased permeability of blood vessels and alteration in osmotic pressures (Settle, 1996). Oedema is at its greatest 1–3 hours after the injury. A gradual decrease in tissue perfusion, at its lowest 12–24 hours after injury, causes ischaemia (Settle, 1996). White blood cells are attracted to the area to begin the process of wound healing. However, the ability of the body to heal itself depends on the depth and extent of the burn.

Systemic pathophysiological effects of a burn injury

An extensive burn injury will have a systemic effect upon the victim, resulting in shock. Advances in the identification, understanding and treatment of these systemic effects have increased the survival rates of burned patients.

The signs and symptoms of shock include:

- *hypotension*: because of fluid loss to oedema and reduced cardiac output
- *cool, clammy, pale skin*: caused by peripheral vasoconstriction (peripheral shutdown)
- *sweating*: sympathetic stimulation and increased adrenaline
- *reduced urine output* caused by hypotension
- *altered mental state* owing to cerebral hypoxia
- *altered pulse*: weak because of hypotension, tachycardic because of increased adrenaline
- *reduced blood pressure*: blood pressure may be maintained for a while because of the compensatory mechanism of peripheral shutdown, but eventually it will fall because of the massive volume loss (Leveridge, 1991)
- *thirst*: caused by fluid loss
- *tachypnoea*: caused by acidosis
- *vomiting*: because of gastric dilation and reduced splanchnic blood flow (Leveridge, 1991).

(Cook, 2002)

Effects upon the skin

We often take for granted the vital part the skin plays in the protection and balance of the other bodily systems. However, once there is major trauma to the skin, the loss of its function becomes only too apparent.

Functions of the skin include:

- maintaining body temperature
- providing a barrier against micro-organisms
- protection from the sun
- sensation
- electrolyte balance
- waterproofing
- synthesis of vitamin D
- the provision of identity.

The most immediate effect of losing an intact skin is fluid loss. An extensive burn injury will result in a massive loss of body fluids, via bleeding and wound exudate. This loss of fluid from the burn injury causes the majority of the other systemic effects.

During the later stages of recovery after a burn injury, that is, once the wounds have healed, the resultant scarring will continue to cause the survivor difficulties not least because of the appearance and cosmesis of the scarred tissue. The scar tissue will be sensitive to sunlight, will need regular moisturizing, may remain fragile and prone to breakdown, and could contract, potentially causing loss of joint motion. Both physiotherapists and occupational therapists play an important role in the care of scar tissue (*see* Chapter 5).

Effects upon the vascular system

Direct trauma to the local vascular supply will occur from a burn injury. If there is full skin thickness tissue loss, the local vascular supply will be blocked because of the development of thrombi and vasoconstriction. Perfusion is reduced, resulting in tissue necrosis (Trofino, 1991). After a partial skin thickness injury the normal flow of blood will be restored within 24–48 hours; however, following a full skin thickness burn injury this process may take up to 3 weeks (Trofino, 1991).

A proportion of red blood cells may also be destroyed (haemolysis) in the area of trauma (Wilson, 2002) and those that remain can become fragile and prone to formation of thrombi because of the increased viscosity of the blood (Trofino, 1991). This haemolysis and reduction in the lifespan of the red blood cells will reduce the patient's haemoglobin levels. The immediate transfusion of blood has been shown to be of little value as, despite this, the haemolysis and fragility of red blood cells continues for the first few days after trauma (Harvey Kemble and Lamb, 1987).

Because of the massive loss of plasma after an extensive burn injury, the concentration of red blood cells in the circulation rises (raised haematocrit). The resultant increased blood viscosity further inhibits tissue perfusion as blood flow is slowed, particularly in the fine peripheral capillaries (Harvey Kemble and Lamb, 1984).

Key point

Tissue perfusion is reduced because of:
- increased haemoconcentration
- reduced cardiac output
- increased oxygen consumption
- haemolysis
- microthrombi
- reduced ventilation (inhalation injury or pulmonary oedema)

(Settle, 1996).

Effects upon the nervous system

At the site of the injury, there may be physical or hypoxic damage to the peripheral nerves. This is most commonly apparent after an electrical burn injury.

Key point

Summary of systemic effects of a major burn injury:
- fluid loss, via wound exudate and interstitial oedema
- reduced cardiac output
- reduced peripheral blood flow
- increased viscosity of blood
- direct trauma to the vasculature, including blood cells
- reduced pulmonary function
- reduced immunity
- reduced renal function
- fat and skeletal muscle catabolism
- gastric ulceration.

(Williams and Phillips, 1996)

Assessment of the burn wound

When assessing the tissue damage after a burn injury, the extent of the trauma and the depth of the tissue loss must be established to ensure that the victim receives adequate resuscitation and treatment. Although estimates of these factors can be made immediately following the injury, a definitive assessment can only take place once the inflammatory responses of the tissues (*see* Chapter 1) have started to diminish, that is, approximately 48 hours later.

Initially, there will be a marked amount of erythema around a burn injury that, on examination, may be judged as superficial skin loss, but that will eventually subside, revealing undamaged tissue. In addition, some areas of burn that initially appear deep will recover over the first couple of days and be classed as partial skin thickness loss instead. However, the opposite may also be true: areas that initially appear superficial may develop to reveal a deeper injury. Rouge et al. (1994) recommended that electrical burns should be reassessed 72 hours after injury, and found that burns continue to evolve over this period of time before stabilizing.

Extent of injury

There are a number of ways to calculate the extent of a burn injury. This is normally stated as a percentage of the total body surface area. The simplest method of calculating the size of small areas of trauma is to take the size of the volar aspect of the patient's hand to represent 1% of the total body surface area and then to estimate how many of these it would take to cover the affected area. However, Sheridan et al. (1995) demonstrated that when assessing irregular shaped burns, a more accurate method was

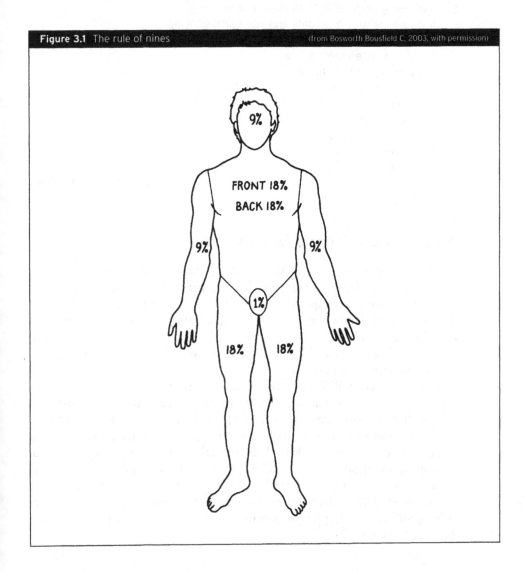

Figure 3.1 The rule of nines   (from Bosworth Bousfield C, 2003, with permission)

to use the size of the patient's palm to represent 0.5% of the total body surface area. An even more accurate method of calculating the size of a burn injury is to use the 'rule of nines'. For this method, the body is divided into percentages (Figure 3.1) and these are used to estimate the total body surface area that is injured.

Depth of injury

The depth of the burn injury will depend upon the following:

- the temperature of the burning agent or the concentration of the chemical
- the duration of exposure
- the method of injury, for example an electrical burn will probably be more severe
- the site of injury, for example the dorsum of hand only has thin cover therefore injury will be deeper.

There are a number of ways to evaluate the depth of a burn injury, but assessment depends on the experience of the assessor. The initial assessment should be reassessed regularly as the injury will change after the immediate trauma.

In order to classify the depth of burn injury, the extent of tissue loss is noted. Different terminology may be used in different burns units, leading to confusion for newer members of staff. Table 3.1 attempts to clarify the terminology used. Figure 3.2 also demonstrates the depths of burn injuries.

Table 3.1 Classification of depth of burn

Superficial burn	First degree	Loss of the most superficial layer of the skin, that is the epidermis
Superficial partial thickness	Second degree (superficial)	Basal membrane partially destroyed, some loss of dermis
Deep partial thickness or deep dermal	Second degree (deep)	Basal membrane completely destroyed, significant loss of dermis
Full thickness	Third degree	Loss of epidermis and dermis, deeper subcutaneous tissues also damaged e.g. fascia or muscle

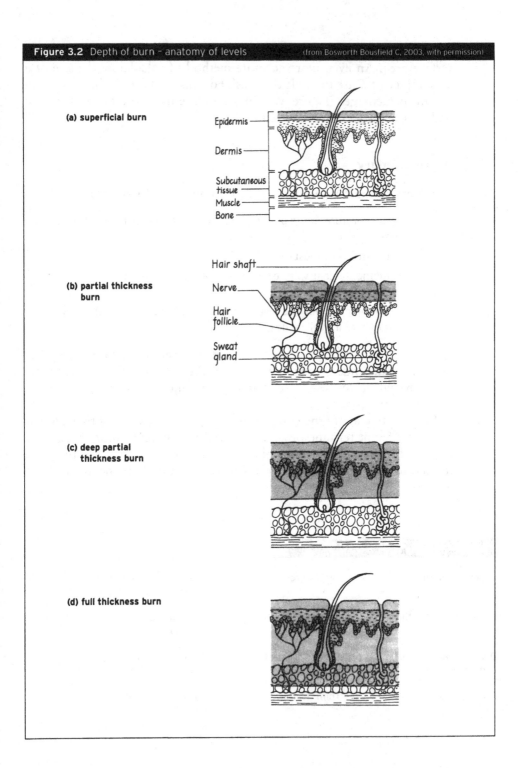

Figure 3.2 Depth of burn – anatomy of levels   (from Bosworth Bousfield C, 2003, with permission)

Assessment of burn depth by observation:

- a superficial burn will appear bright pink
- a partial thickness burn will appear pink, wet and may have blisters
- a full thickness burn could appear black and charred if sustained from flame or electricity, but the bed of the wound will be white and waxy because of the lack of circulation.

Assessment of burn depth by sensation:

- a superficial burn will be very painful due to the exposure of nerve endings
- a partial thickness burn will have some areas that are painful but other areas that are sensate but dulled
- a full thickness burn will initially be pain-free, even to the application of a pin-prick, because of the destruction of the nerve endings.

Assessment of burn depth by capillary refill:

- a superficial burn will blanch with pressure but capillary refill will be rapid owing to the inflammatory response vasodilating the blood vessels in the area
- a partial thickness burn will blanch with pressure but the capillary response may be sluggish and delayed because of damage to the blood vessels
- a full thickness burn will not blanch nor will capillary flow be evident because of the destruction of blood vessels.

Assessment of burn depth by healing:

- a superficial burn takes up to 5 days to heal
- a partial thickness burn takes 3 weeks to 1 month to heal if it is superficial and from 30 days to months if it is deep dermal
- a full thickness burn will not heal independently unless it is very small.

Assessment of burn depth by scarring:

- scarring after a partial thickness burn depends on the depth, the deeper the burn the greater the incidence of scarring
- scarring after full thickness burns can be minimized by the use of skin grafting.

Assessment of depth by laser doppler scan:

This is a relatively recent development in the assessment of the depth of a wound. The device measures wound perfusion and produces a digital image. Superficial burns have a very high perfusion, whereas the perfusion of deep burns is markedly reduced (Niazi et al., 1993).

References

Cook D (2002) Classification of burn trauma. In: C Bosworth Bousfield Burns Trauma: Management and Nursing Care (second edition). London: Whurr Publishers.

Harvey Kemble JV, Lamb BE (1984) Plastic Surgical and Burns Nursing. London: Baillière Tindall.

Harvey Kemble JV, Lamb BE (1987) Practical Burns Management. London: Hodder & Stoughton.

Leveridge A (1991) Therapy for the Burn Patient. London: Chapman & Hall.

Niazi ZBM, Essex TJH, Papini R, Scott D, McLean NR, Black MJM (1993) New laser Doppler scanner: a valuable adjunct in burn depth assessment. Burns 19: 485–9.

Rouge D, Polynice A, Grolleau JL, Nicoulet B, Chavoin JP, Costagliola M (1994) Histological assessment of low voltage electrical burns: experimental study with pig skin. Journal of Burn Care and Rehabilitation 15: 328-34.

Settle JAD (1996) Principles and Practice of Burns Management. London: Churchill Livingstone.

Sheridan RL, Petras L, Basha G, Salvo P, Cifrino C, Hinson M et al. (1995) Planimetry study of the percent of body surface represented by the hand and palm: sizing irregular burns is more accurately done with the palm. Journal of Burn Care and Rehabilitation 16: 605-6.

Trofino RB (1991) Nursing Care of the Burn-injured Patient. Philadelphia, PA: FA Davies.

Williams WG, Phillips LG (1996) Pathophysiology of the burn wound. In: DN Herndon Total Burn Care. London: WB Saunders, chapter 7.

Wilson DI (2002) Management in the first 48 hours. In: C Bosworth Bousfield Burns Trauma: Management and Nursing Care (second edition). London: Whurr Publishers.

Chapter 4

Principles of plastic surgery

Introduction

Reconstruction of the hand presents surgeons with a difficult problem. As far as is achievable the skin coverage that is used must be extensible, sensate and cosmetically acceptable. In addition, the functional units (muscles, tendons, joints and nerves) within the hand must be rebuilt or replaced. The aims of plastic surgery are to:

- achieve wound closure
- prevent infection
- re-establish the properties and function of an intact skin
- reconstruct tissue after trauma or previous elective procedures.

The reconstructive ladder

The reconstructive options available to plastic surgeons can be viewed hierarchically. In fact, they are commonly known as the 'reconstructive ladder' (Figure 4.1). The first step towards reconstruction may simply be conservative wound management with dressings, and the most complex option available is a free-flap reconstruction. When deciding upon an appropriate method of reconstruction plastic surgeons must consider the extent of missing tissue and the structures that have been affected (Ranelli et al., 2000). If possible, wound closure should be obtained by conservative methods, if not then direct closure by suture is employed. If there is a risk of increased skin tension with direct closure or if there is skin loss, a skin graft may be necessary. If a skin graft would not survive because of an avascular bed a more extensive reconstructive procedure may be required, starting with a simple skin flap and extending to a free flap depending upon the individual situation (Davies, 1996).

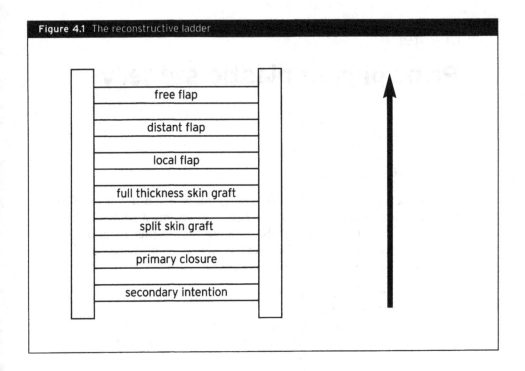

Figure 4.1 The reconstructive ladder

Surgery for burned patients

Surgical intervention for burned patients is not normally indicated until the depth of the burn has been established some 48 hours after injury (*see* Chapter 3). The two exceptions to this are: the early excision of obviously necrotic tissue if the patient is becoming septic; and if escharotomy is needed. An escharotomy is the surgical division of necrotic tissue (eschar) that is the result of a full thickness burn. The procedure is needed if a full thickness burn is circumferential around a limb, the neck or chest. Eschar is thick burnt tissue that cannot expand as skin does, therefore if it is circumferential it will form a tourniquet as the limb becomes oedematous, decreasing perfusion to the distal extremities and causing ischaemia.

Partial thickness burn injuries may result in blistering of the skin. If these blisters are small they can be left in place as the skin will heal beneath them. However, if the blisters are large and cross joints, they will limit range of motion and function. Therefore, the surface of these blisters should be excised (deroofed) and the resultant wound cleaned and dressed.

Once the depth of the burn has been established, the experienced burns surgeon will be able to decide the most appropriate intervention. It may be that no surgical intervention is indicated – a superficial partial thickness burn will heal with conservative treatment only (that is, dressings) in 10 days to 3 weeks, unless it becomes infected (Leveridge, 1991). Deep partial thickness and full thickness burns require surgical intervention. Surgery should take place within the first 5 days after injury to prevent the development of infection (Leveridge, 1991). If a wound becomes infected the depth of the tissue loss can be extended.

Secondary intention

Conservative management of wounds

Surgical intervention may not be needed for wound healing. If a wound is of such a size that it will heal naturally with the aid and protection of dressings then this is the simplest and cheapest route. It is, however, essential that an experienced nurse monitors the wound regularly to ensure that healing is progressing as it should and that the most appropriate dressing is being used. There are an enormous amount of dressings available that are specifically designed for the treatment of different wounds. They are too numerous to mention in this text but they all aim to create an environment that aids the body's natural healing process and prevents infection. This method of wound closure is often termed 'secondary healing' or 'healing by secondary intention', where a wound is allowed to heal spontaneously. Primary wound closure occurs when the wound is directly closed and sutured (as will be discussed later).

Tangential excision

An open wound that requires surgical intervention for closure may first require tangential excision. The surgeon gradually and progressively debrides the surface of the wound until the necrotic tissue is removed and only healthy tissue remains. Healthy tissue bleeds, therefore, after debridement the wound bed should be bleeding. If this does not happen the surgeon will need to continue the debridement. It is essential that all the necrotic tissue is removed and the wound bed is bleeding before the next stage of surgery. Bailie (1997) noted that early tangential excision of wounds aimed to:

- increase the rate of healing
- reduce infection
- reduce the severity of scarring.

However, tangential excision should not be performed without precautions against excessive blood loss and infection (Bailie, 1997). Techniques that reduce the amount of blood loss during surgery include:

- elevation
- tourniquet
- compression
- diathermy
- ligation of vessels
- adrenaline – either topical or subcutaneous
- homeostatic agents, such as thrombin.

Fascial excision

If the injury is obviously full thickness and therefore preservation of the dermis is inappropriate, fascial excision (debridement to the fascia, removing all skin layers and subcutaneous fat, and into the underlying tissues) is necessary. Fascial excision can be performed much more quickly than tangential excision and the amount of blood loss is significantly reduced. When skin grafts are applied after fascial excision they usually take very well, owing to the highly vascular bed. However, the cosmetic result is poor because of the depth of the excision, which leaves an indentation. Fascial excision is most appropriate for unstable or elderly patients who require a shorter anaesthetic.

Direct or primary closure

If a wound is of such a size that it can be closed directly without producing undue tension at the wound site this should be done, as it will produce the best cosmetic result, that is, a thin line of scar tissue. When judging the tension at a directly closed wound the surgeon must allow for the development of oedema (Roehr et al., 1997). Increased tension at a wound site can cause:

- delayed healing
- stretched unsightly scarring
- dehiscence of the wound.

Quaba (1995) noted that breakdown of directly closed wounds was caused by:

- poor surgical technique
- rough handling of tissues
- infection
- inadequate circulation.

After direct closure, a wound should be covered with a non-adherent dressing. Sutures should be removed from the hand after 7 days to 2 weeks. Absorbable suture materials are more appropriate for children to avoid sutures having to be removed later on (Roehr et al., 1997).

Delayed primary closure

If a wound is contaminated, or an infection is suspected, primary closure is detrimental to tissue healing. Thorough irrigation with saline, adequate debridement and the prescription of systemic antibiotics is appropriate, followed by the wound being left open for a few days to monitor it and allow drainage (Quaba, 1995). Once the wound looks clean and healthy, it can be closed.

Skin grafts

A skin graft is the transposition of skin from one area of the body to another. The skin graft is separated from its original blood supply and therefore requires a highly vascular recipient bed to thrive. There are a number of methods of grafting onto a debrided wound to obtain closure:

- autograft (own skin)
- allograft (donor skin)
- heterograft or xenografts (animal skin)
- cultured skin
- artificial skin.

Settle (1996) described the criteria that should be met before early tangential excision and grafting of burn injuries:

- a firm diagnosis of a deep loss of tissue should be established
- the patient needs to be systemically fit enough to have surgery
- the patient should not have any coagulation abnormalities
- there should be sufficient donor sites available
- the wound should be clear of streptococcus (Cason, 1981).

Autograft

Uninjured skin is taken from the patient and used to cover the wound. The graft is often called a 'split skin graft' as the depth of skin harvested is split through the dermis. Split skin grafts can be thin, intermediate or thick depending upon the depth of dermis that is harvested (McGregor and McGregor, 2000). The thinner the graft, the less nutrition it requires and therefore the more likely it is to take (Ranelli et al., 2000). The thicker the section of dermis that is taken with the graft, the less the graft will contract subsequently (Ranelli et al., 2000). Before applying an autograft it may be meshed to allow wound exudate and blood to drain through it. If this were not done a haematoma could develop beneath the graft and this would result in graft failure (Brcic, 1990). If there is a limited supply of uninjured skin because of the extent of the injury the skin may be stretched or expanded once it has been meshed, to cover a larger surface area of the wound (Bailie, 1997). Stretching meshed skin creates a 'string vest' appearance to the graft. Once it is laid onto the wound, the holes will be filled in by epithelialization (*see* Chapter 1). Unfortunately, if the meshed skin does need to be stretched, the resultant scar tissue maintains the 'string vest' pattern so it is unacceptable to use this technique in cosmetic areas, that is, the face and hands. Skin grafts are secured to the recipient site by staples, sutures, glue or just laid over wound (Roehr et al., 1997).

Kim and Kim (1999) reported the advantages and disadvantages of meshing autografts:

- *Advantages*: can cover a large area; will contour to fit irregular surfaces; permits draining of exudate and blood; increases surface area of edges from which epithelialization can take place.
- *Disadvantages*: a large proportion of the wound heals by secondary intention, therefore the scarring is more likely to contract; cosmetic result is poor.

The most common donor site is a patient's thigh; however, almost any part of the body may be used if necessary, although cosmetic areas such as the face should be avoided. The depth of skin taken from the donor site should leave a superficial or superficial partial thickness wound. The exposure of nerve endings in the donor site wound causes patients to report a significant amount of pain – commonly patients report that the donor site is more troublesome to them than the original injury (Ranelli et al., 2000). The donor site will heal spontaneously in 10–14 days, at which stage it may be reused if necessary. As the lower portions of the dermis are left intact after the split skin graft is harvested the epithelial structures will also be intact and aid epithelialization (*see* Chapter 1).

The skin graft should 'take' in 5 days and will provide permanent covering of the injury. However, if it is not placed over bleeding, healthy tissue it will fail because the body is unable to vascularize the graft (McGregor and McGregor, 2000), for example insufficiently debrided wound, infected wound, bare bone, exposed cartilage or tendon. Post-operatively, a dressing is applied to create pressure over the graft to limit haematoma formation and to immobilize the body part to prevent shearing forces disrupting the graft. On very mobile parts of the body, such as the hand, it may be necessary to splint the surrounding joints to ensure immobility. The first dressing check will be made between 3 and 5 days after the procedure.

If skin grafts are not used immediately after harvesting, or if extra skin has been harvested in case of graft failure, it may be stored at a temperature of 4°C for 2–3 weeks (Bailie, 1997). Grafting may need to be delayed if the wound bed bleeds profusely after debridement; the application of a graft to this type of wound would certainly fail because of the formation of haematomas.

Roehr et al. (1997) reported the advantages and disadvantages of skin grafts as follows:

- *Advantages*: readily available; easy to harvest; can be stored for up to 3 weeks in a refrigerator.
- *Disadvantage*: cosmetic defect; possible mechanically vulnerable donor site; altered pigmentation.

Quaba (1995) added further disadvantages:

- contraction
- lack of growth in children
- abnormal pigmentation
- lack of durability.

Monitoring the graft

The skin graft can be nursed exposed or covered. If covered, it is usually dressed with layers of non-adherent paraffin gauze, dry gauze and bandages. If left exposed, nursing staff must watch for signs of infection, haematoma or blistering. If the graft is displaced within the first few hours post-operatively it can be re-aligned. The benefits of exposing a graft are that it can be observed and accessed easily, any displacement can be identified and rectified immediately. The benefits of dressing a graft are that patients are more mobile, the pressure exerted by the dressings will prevent haematomas, the graft is protected from direct trauma and the patient does not have to see the graft in the initial stages of healing (Harvey Kemble and Lamb, 1984).

Allograft

Cadaver skin, or skin donated from a family member, may be applied to the wound. However, this type of graft will only 'take' for a short period, about 3 weeks, before being rejected. Whilst in place the graft will act like normal skin and provide protection from infection and fluid loss. It is an ideal dressing for the wound and may buy time whilst further autograft donor sites are recovering (Leveridge, 1991).

Heterograft (xenografts)

Porcine skin may be used to cover a burn wound, although it will also be rejected after 4 days (Harvey Kemble and Lamb, 1984).

Cultured skin

A few centres in the UK offer a skin culturing service; however, the process is slow and expensive and is not used often. Munster et al. (1990) compared the use of cultured epidermis with conventional autografts to cover extensive burn injuries and found that there were no significant differences between the two groups in length of hospital stay, number of operations or cost. However, these researchers did note that it took 3 weeks to culture the skin and that because of the fragility of the grafts, rehabilitation (including exercise and pressure garment therapy) needed to be delayed.

Artificial skin

The most recent development in burns surgery is the development of artificial skin. This was initially used in 1980 and is now commonly used in USA but is still currently being researched in the UK. A dermal matrix made from bovine collagen and shark cartilage (Tompkins and Burke, 1996) is placed on the debrided burn wound. It is covered with a silicone layer that provides wound homeostasis. This remains in place for 3 weeks then the silicone layer is removed and a very thin split skin autograft is harvested to cover the wound. It is claimed that the artificial skin provides a biodegradable template into which the body can regenerate dermal tissue. Because of the more structured dermal regeneration, it is claimed that the collagen does not contract as much, therefore skin and joint contractures are avoided.

Sheridan et al. (1994) reported an 80% success rate when using artificial skin. Scarring, contracture, growth in children and cosmesis were found to compare favourably with autografted areas. In fact, Sheridan et al. (1994) claimed that none of their subjects developed significant joint contractures. In a randomized trial by Heimbach et al. (1988), unsurprisingly, donor site skin thickness was found to be significantly less for patients who had artificial skin grafts compared with traditional autografts, and donor site healing took on average 4 days less. Heimbach et al. (1988) also claimed that cosmesis, scarring and function was improved with artificial skin coverage.

Full thickness skin grafts

In burns care these grafts are more commonly used as a secondary procedure once the patient is stable and has recovered from the injury (Bailie, 1997). The full thickness of the skin (epidermis and full thickness of dermis) is harvested and used to reconstruct areas (such as the first web space) after release of skin contractures. Full thickness skin grafts are less likely to contract and provide a more acceptable appearance and colour match (Ranelli et al., 2000). The most common donor site for a full thickness skin graft is the groin. The full thickness graft is not meshed, therefore it must be protected from haematoma formation to ensure a good 'take' by the application of pressure to the graft. A bolus of cotton wool, foam or gauze is tied over the graft using the sutures that secure the graft into the defect (McGregor and McGregor, 2000), this technique is called a 'tie over'. A further pressure dressing over the top of the tie over creates added pressure and help to immobilize the body part and prevent shearing forces being applied by motion.

Despite the advantages of resistance to contraction, the ability to grow with children, and the provision of good texture and pigmentation (Harvey Kemble and Lamb, 1984; Quaba, 1995), full thickness skin grafts need a very clean, highly vascular recipient bed to survive (Quaba, 1995). They also take less readily than split skin grafts, do not regain much sensation (Harvey Kemble and Lamb, 1984) and have a high incidence of hypersensitivity (Roehr et al., 1997).

Graft 'take'

This is the common terminology used to express that the skin graft has been successful. Ranelli et al. (2000) described the process of graft take in three phases:

- *Serum imbibition* (24–48 hours): formation of fibrin layer and diffusion of fluid from the wound bed.
- *Inosculation* (day 3): capillary budding from the wound bed up into the base of the graft.
- *Capillary in-growth and remodelling.*

Graft failure may be caused by:

- inadequate blood supply to the wound bed
- movement of the graft
- collection of fluid (for example, haematoma) beneath the graft
- infection, in particular some strains of haemolytic streptococcus will cause graft failure.

(Harvey Kemble and Lamb, 1984)

Kim and Kim (1999) add to this list the actual properties of the graft itself, that is to say, the more vascular the area from which the graft is harvested, the greater the chance of its survival.

Flaps

Reconstructive surgery with flaps is not as new as we might believe. Evidence of the use of flaps can be found in ancient India and Persia (Roehr et al., 1997). The historical development of flap surgery is fascinating but unfortunately out of the scope of this text. Development of plastic surgery techniques began after the Second World War, intiated by the magnitude of trauma suffered, and has progressed since then. It was not until as recently as the 1970s and 1980s that free-flap surgery was achievable, owing to advances in microsurgery, and tubed flaps became obsolete.

If a wound bed is avascular, a skin graft will not take over it. Unlike a skin graft, a flap contains its own vasculature within its substance (McGregor and McGregor, 2000) and is therefore suitable to cover an avascular wound. Tissues over which a skin graft will not take are:

- bone without periosteum
- tendon without paratenon
- cartilage without perichondrium (Singer et al., 1995).

However, flaps are not only used to cover difficult wounds, they can also be used to release contractures, for example 'Z-plasty', to provide subcutaneous tissue to fill areas, provide wear and tear properties and to reconstruct areas of deficit. There are numerous types of flaps reported in the literature; the different types of flap can be categorized according to their:

- vascularity, for example random or axial
- anatomical composition
- method of relocation.

Flap vascularity

To understand flap construction it is vital to understand the anatomical vascularity of tissues. The major blood vessels usually lie deep in the tissues; they emit branches that enter tissue groups, such as muscle. As the vessels branch within the muscle they send perforator vessels up through the overlying fascia and into the subdermal plexus, which is also supplied directly from cutaneous vessels (Quaba, 1995).

Random pattern flaps

This is a flap of skin that is not raised on any particular blood vessel, but survives on the subdermal plexus of vessels alone (Singer et al., 1995). Therefore, the size of the flap is limited to ensure that the most distal portions do not become ischaemic. The skin flap remains in continuity with its origin by its base. Examples of random pattern flaps are the Z-plasty, V–Y advancement flap, rotation flap and transposition flap.

Z-plasty

If skin contractures develop, for example in the web spaces between digits or along the volar aspect of a digit, they can be released and reconstructed with a full thickness skin graft (as above) or, if the contracture is narrow, the surgical technique of Z-plasty can be used. This is the transposition of two triangular skin flaps that are drawn on the line of contracture in the shape of a 'Z' – hence the name. By transposing the two flaps, the distance along the length of the contracture is increased (McGregor and McGregor, 2000) (*see* Figure 4.2). The angle of the flaps is usually set at 60° (Roehr et al., 1997) and the central part of the Z follows the line of contracture. As the flaps are raised and the contracted tissue released, the tension is also released, therefore allowing lengthening in the line of contracture (McGregor and McGregor, 2000). The two triangular flaps are then transposed to produce a horizontal scar line as opposed to a vertical one in an attempt to prevent recurrence of the contracture. The Z-plasty technique not only increases the vertical distance of an area but also results in a decrease in the horizontal distance (McGregor and McGregor, 2000). The Z-plasty may be modified by the surgeon for individual patients' needs by slightly altering the size and shape of the flaps raised or by using multiple Z-plasties (McGregor and McGregor, 2000).

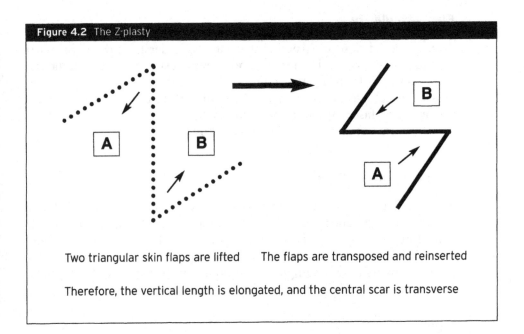

Figure 4.2 The Z-plasty

Two triangular skin flaps are lifted   The flaps are transposed and reinserted

Therefore, the vertical length is elongated, and the central scar is transverse

Axial flaps

In certain areas of the body flaps can be raised upon specific blood vessels, allowing the skin flap to be lifted on a narrow pedicle. Because of the greater certainty of the flap perfusion with this technique, it is more resilient and more likely to survive. Examples of axial flaps include the following.

- *Groin flap*: based the on superficial circumflex iliac artery, this is particularly useful in covering the dorsum of the hand (*see* below).
- *Delto-pectoral flap*: based on the perforating vessels of the internal mammary artery.
- *Forehead flap*: based on the anterior branch of the superficial temporal artery.

Flap anatomical composition

Definition by composition (*see* Figure 4.3):

- *Skin flap*: epidermis, dermis and superficial fascia.
- *Fasciocutaneous flap*: epidermis, dermis and both superficial plus deep fascia.
- *Muscle flap*: muscle belly without overlying structures, the muscle may be covered with a split skin graft once it has been repositioned, this prevents donor site skin loss (Harvey Kemble and Lamb, 1984).
- *Myocutaneous flap*: muscle belly with the overlying skin, the skin's blood supply originates from perforator vessels from the underlying muscle (Harvey Kemble and Lamb, 1984) therefore if the flap is raised, maintaining the perfusion to the muscle, the skin will survive.
- *Osseous flap*: bone.
- *Osseomyocutaneous flap*: bone, muscle and skin.
- *Composite flap*: this may include a number of different tissues, such as skin, fascia, muscle and bone. These flaps are used to repair defects (Harvey Kemble and Lamb, 1984), for example a radial forearm flap can be used with part of the radius to reconstruct the jaw because of the hairless skin and colour match (Mankani and Pribaz, 1999).

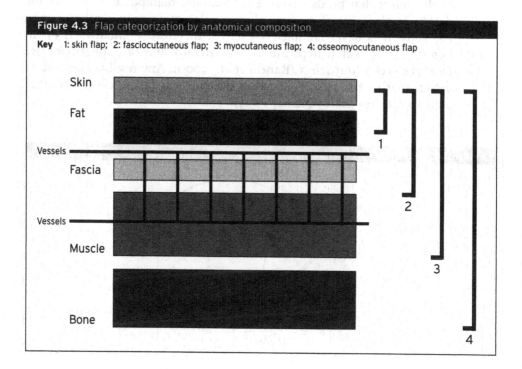

Figure 4.3 Flap categorization by anatomical composition

Key 1: skin flap; 2: fasciocutaneous flap; 3: myocutaneous flap; 4: osseomyocutaneous flap

Fasciocutaneous flaps rely on the fact that perforating vessels supply a vascular plexus superficial to the deep fascia (Davies, 1996). Therefore including the fascia with the perforating vessel means that large flaps can be raised (Davies, 1996). Fasciocutaneous flaps are of particular use in covering defects in the limbs as they can either be raised proximally or distally (Davies, 1996).

Myocutaneous flaps are based on a major vessel that enters a muscle but also supports its overlying skin. This allows a large muscle flap, plus its skin, to be raised and rotated in any direction as long as the vessel remains in continuity (Davies, 1996).

Relocation of flaps

Definition by method of transfer, 'flaps can be classed as either local or distant depending upon the site of the donor area in relation to the defect' (Quaba, 1995).

Local flaps

Rotation or transposition flap (*see* Figure 4.4 and Figure 4.5): tissue local to the defect that needs covering is lifted and manipulated to cover the defect. At all stages of the procedure the flap remains in continuity with the body, it is never completely excised, therefore vascularity is maintained. Transposition flaps are moved laterally and rotational flaps are rotated to cover the defect (Ranelli et al., 2000). Any resulting secondary defect, that is, the area from where the flap was taken, can be covered with a split skin graft (Quaba, 1995).

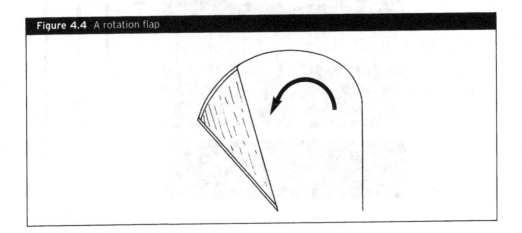

Figure 4.4 A rotation flap

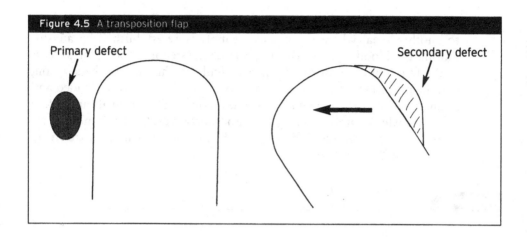

Figure 4.5 A transposition flap

Advancement flaps: after being undermined, tissue is moved directly forward to cover the defect, without the need for any manipulation (laterally or by rotation), for example V–Y flaps (Ranelli et al., 2000), which can be used to cover fingertip injuries without the digit length having to be reduced (*see* Figure 4.6).

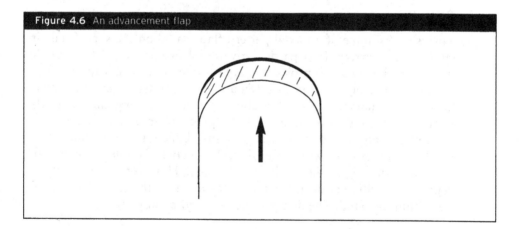

Figure 4.6 An advancement flap

Distant flaps

Pedicled flap: tissue is transferred to another area of the body, but a vascular attachment is always maintained (McGregor and McGregor, 2000). The distance a pedicled flap can be transported depends on the length of the pedicle.

Free flap: tissue is completely separated from the body and transferred to another area, where the vascular supply is re-established by anastomosing the blood vessels (McGregor and McGregor, 2000). The success of the free flap depends on the microvascular techniques of the surgeon, and the procedure allows axial and myocutaneous flaps to be divided and re-anastomosed at recipient sites (Davies, 1996). The survival rate of free tissue transfer is more than 95%, with almost 100% of the more commonly used procedures done by experienced plastic surgeons surviving (Buntic and Buncke, 1999).

Key point

Flaps are categorized according to:

- vascularity
- composition
- method of relocation

Common flaps used to reconstruct the hand

Groin flap

This is an example of an axial pattern flap, based on the superficial circumflex iliac artery. It is particularly useful in covering defects of the dorsum of the hand as it provides a large amount of cosmetically good tissue on a relatively short pedicle (Figure 4.7). The flap is stitched to the hand and remains in place for about 3 weeks. During this time, the patient's arm is supported using a sling or collar and cuff, and tape secured around the arm and chest prevents abduction of the limb, which would create tension within the flap. The patient is able to move and exercising the digits should be encouraged. However, because of the dependent position of the hand, the disadvantage of the groin flap is oedema within the hand. The donor site can be closed directly.

Cross-finger flap

This is an example of a local flap that is raised on the dorsal surface of a digit and attached to the palmar aspect or tip of an adjacent digit (McGregor and McGregor, 2000) (*see* Figure 4.8). The flap remains attached to its origin for 2–3 weeks before it is separated. During this time the patient is encouraged to maintain mobility of unaffected digits or

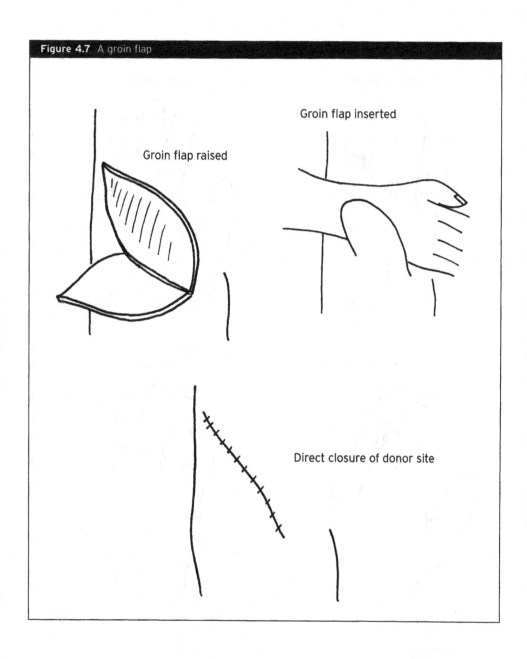

Figure 4.7 A groin flap

Groin flap inserted

Groin flap raised

Direct closure of donor site

joints whilst protecting the flap from tension. The donor site is closed by a split skin graft, which will 'take' so long as the paratenon of the extensor mechanism has been preserved during harvesting of the flap (McGregor and McGregor, 2000).

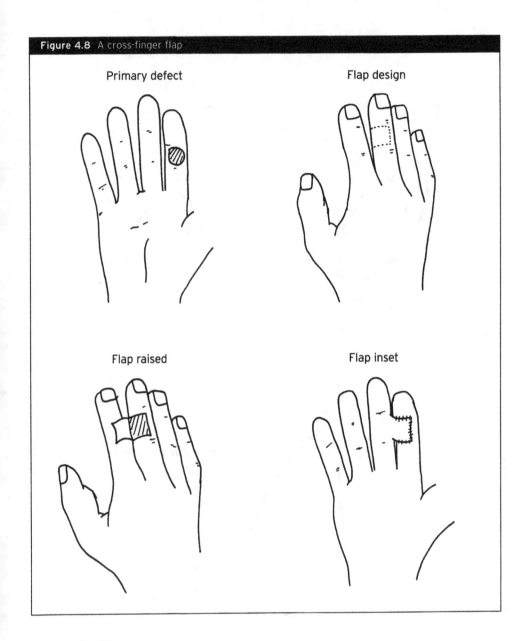

Figure 4.8 A cross-finger flap

V-Y flaps

This is an example of an advancement flap that is of particular use in covering a fingertip injury, yet maintaining sensation. A V-shaped flap is raised in the pulp tissue, preserving the neurovascular supply, and advanced distally. The proximal portion of the donor area is approximated and sutured, thereby creating a Y shape (*see* Figure 4.9).

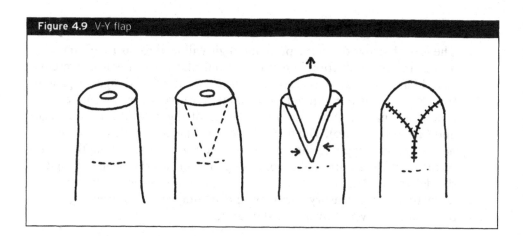

Figure 4.9 V-Y flap

Thenar flap

Another local flap that is useful in covering fingertip injuries is the thenar flap. The flap is raised from the palmar skin and the finger is flexed to meet the flap (*see* Figure 4.10). Disadvantages of thenar flaps are the risk of PIP joint contracture, as the flap is not divided for 2 weeks, and insensitivity. It should be possible to close the donor site directly.

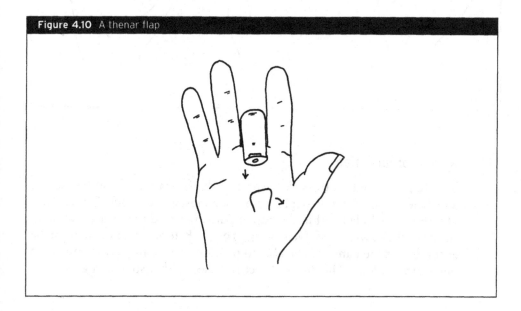

Figure 4.10 A thenar flap

Neurovascular island flap

The loss of sensation to the pulp of a digit will lead to disuse of that digit and therefore a reduction in hand function. The aim of the neurovascular island flap is to restore sensation to the tip of an injured digit. A proportion of previously uninjured pulp tissue is raised from a relatively less functional digit, such as the ulnar border of the ring finger (McGregor and McGregor, 2000). The flap is raised on a pedicle, which preserves the neurovascular supply to the skin. The pedicle is dissected along the length of the digit then tunnelled across the palm and up the recipient digit to the defect (*see* Figure 4.11). After a period of adjustment, most patients learn to use the sensory recovery and no longer disuse the digit. The donor site is covered by a split skin graft.

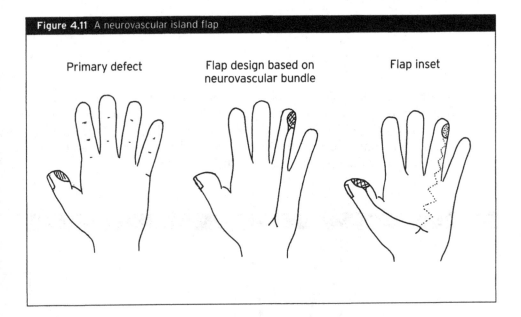

Figure 4.11 A neurovascular island flap

Primary defect   Flap design based on   Flap inset
                      neurovascular bundle

Radial forearm flap

This flap is raised on the volar aspect of the forearm and can be used as a pedicle flap or as a free flap. As a pedicled fasciocutaneous flap the radial artery is included within the flap and it is reversed to cover distal hand trauma (Weinzweig and Weinzweig, 1999). Before elevation it must be ensured that the hand will be able to maintain adequate perfusion via the ulnar artery alone. The donor defect is closed with a split skin graft.

Figure 4.12 A reversed radial forearm flap

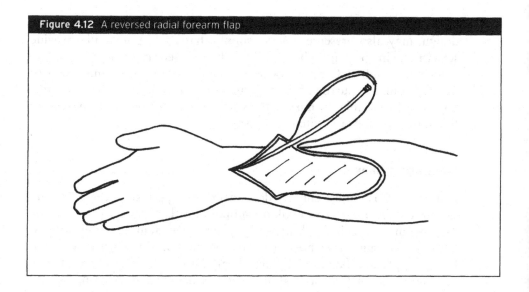

Functional free muscle transfer

If there has been severe loss of musculature of the forearm, causing a significant reduction in hand function, a muscle (such as the gracilis) can be relocated and re-innervated by connecting a motor nerve in the area of injury to the motor nerve of the donor muscle, thereby restoring function (Weinzweig and Weinzweig, 1999).

Delayed flaps

Occasionally, a flap will be raised on three of its four aspects and then re-inserted for a few days to encourage capillary growth into its most distal portion. After this, the flap can be transferred to its recipient site. The aim of this delayed procedure is to enable larger flaps to be used without flap necrosis of the distal portion (Stotland and Kerrigan, 1999).

Innervation of flaps

Local flaps, such as transposition, rotational and advancement flaps, maintain their neurological supply and are therefore sensate. This is particularly beneficial in their use in hand surgery to provide wound coverage whilst preserving sensation (Ranelli et al., 2000). An example of a flap that is specifically designed to restore sensation to a digit is the neurovascular island flap (*see* Figure 4.11 above). Although free flaps, by design, may also preserve a nerve supply that could potentially provide sensation, in practice the quality of this sensation is inadequate (McGregor and McGregor, 2000). Other flaps rely on the ingrowth of nerves from the surrounding uninjured tissue, but the extent of this ingrowth is variable. In muscle flaps it is often preferential to denervate the muscle to prevent twitching spasms.

Monitoring flaps

Flap survival is almost entirely dependent upon perfusion, therefore any significant disruption to the blood supply of a flap will cause its failure. The role of the specialist plastic surgery nurse is vital in the monitoring of flaps in the immediate post-operative period as, if problems with the blood supply to a flap are recognized early, it may be possible to salvage it. Soutar and McGregor (1986) suggested that flap monitoring should continue every half-hour for up to 36 hours. Patients should also be nursed in a room that is kept at a higher temperature than normal; this raised temperature will cause vasodilation of the blood vessels within the flap, thus increasing the blood flow.

Signs of vascular insufficiency

- *Colour:* the colour of the flap should be compared with the donor site, not the area of insertion; it should remain pink (Edwards, 1994). The flap may become dusky blue, demonstrating poor venous drainage, or it may look pale or white, indicating an arterial problem. Although colour monitoring is subjective (Coull and Wylie, 1990), regular monitoring by the same member of nursing staff should permit the early identification of colour change.
- *Temperature:* the flap should remain warm (Edwards, 1994); if it becomes cold a failure in perfusion may be indicated (Anthony, 1997). Conversely, if the flap temperature increases this could be indicative of infection.
- *Texture:* feeling the texture of a flap will inform the nurse of the processes occurring within it. The flap should feel soft (Edwards, 1994); any areas of firmness may indicate the formation of a haematoma (Coull and Wylie, 1990).
- *Blanching:* a delay in capillary refill after the application of momentary pressure could indicate a disruption in perfusion. An acceptable capillary refill time is 1-3 seconds, more than 3 seconds indicates reduced arterial supply, whereas a refill time of less than 1 second may be caused by venous congestion (Edwards, 1994).

Indications of disruption in flap perfusion:
- altered colour
- altered temperature
- altered texture
- excessively slow or fast capillary refill

Causes of vascular insufficiency

- *Hypothermia*: cooling the patient or the flap will cause vasoconstriction (Edwards, 1994).
- *Systemic variation in blood pressure*: hypotension will cause a reduction in arterial flow to the flap, whereas hypertension will cause venous congestion of the flap and an increased risk of emboli (Coull and Wylie, 1990).
- *Kinking*: the blood vessels may be kinked, causing a disruption in blood flow.
- *Tension*: overstretching the flap may occlude the blood vessels; attention should be paid to the position of the flap and the tension of the sutures and drains.
- *Pressure*: too much compression over the flap will decrease its perfusion, attention should be paid to dressings (Edwards, 1994) and splints, etc. Care must also be taken to ensure the patient does not lie directly on the flap or the pedicle (Edwards, 1994).
- *Haematoma*: bleeding within the flap will lead to the development of a haematoma; this will increase flap pressure and reduce perfusion. The insertion of drains will reduce the risk of haematoma formation (Edwards, 1994).
- *Infection*: the release of toxins caused by infection or the accumulation of pus beneath the flap will affect the 'take' (Coull and Wylie, 1990); prophylactic antibiotics may be used as a precaution (Edwards, 1994).
- *Nicotine*: vasospasm and the risk of thrombi is increased, smokers also have a lower haemoglobin level and therefore reduced oxygen-carrying capacity (Coull and Wylie, 1990). Smoking has detrimental effects on cutaneous blood flow, wound healing and therefore flap reconstructive surgery (Reus et al., 1992) and should therefore be restricted after microvascular surgery (van Adrichem et al., 1992).
- *Dehydration*: this will increase blood viscosity and the risk of clotting (Coull and Wylie, 1990).
- *Caffeine*: may cause vasospasm (Bonavita, 1985).

Treatment options include the following.

- Surgical allowance for oedema development: post-operatively the reconstructed area will swell, just as any other traumatized tissue would. If the surgeon does not allow for this oedema when the flap is inserted it could create tension within the flap and reduce perfusion.
- Release of tension or kinking by repositioning (Harvey Kemble and Lamb, 1984).
- Evacuation of haematoma.
- Aid venous return by positioning the flap so that it drains downwards.
- Administer anticoagulants such as heparin or aspirin (Edwards, 1994).
- The use of dextran increases blood flow within the capillaries and decreases viscosity (Harvey Kemble and Lamb, 1984).
- Leeches cause vasodilation and aid vascular decompression by injecting an anticoagulant and ingesting the excess blood (Valauri, 1991). Current estimates on the effectiveness of leeches in rescuing at-risk replanted digits and pedicled flaps is 60–70% (Daane, 1999).
- Re-anastomosis of vessels or vein grafts.

Donor site

Often, the donor site for a skin graft or flap can be overlooked (Ranelli et al., 2000) because of preoccupation with the primary wound. However, donor sites may require intervention to maintain tissue extensibility and scar management, for example the donor site after radial forearm flap can cause secondary complications to hand function if not treated adequately.

When a donor site is selected, the surgeon must consider colour match, hair growth and scar visibility. Quaba (1995) suggests that after trauma, degloved or amputated tissue can be used to reconstruct a defect, for example skin from an amputated digit could be used to cover the stump.

Further plastic surgery procedures

Tissue expansion

Healthy skin can be stretched by inserting a subcutaneous, tissue expander. Over a number of weeks, the expander is gradually filled with saline and as it inflates the overlying skin is stretched. When the expander is removed, the surgeon is able to use the extra skin to cover a defect. Although use of this device is uncommon in coverage of the hand it has been reported by Weinzweig and Weinzweig (1999).

Nerve repair

This is most appropriate after a clean, sharp cut of a nerve (Tonkin, 1997). It is not possible in traction or avulsion injuries as a nerve graft would be necessary if a significant portion of the nerve were missing. Usually, only the epineurium is repaired as, despite attempts at fasicular repair, there is no evidence of better recovery (Nath and Mackinnon, 1999).

Nerve grafting

Nerve grafting simply provides a tube that the injured nerve can grow down (Harvey Kemble and Lamb, 1984). If the axonal buds do not have direction of growth they will grow in a haphazard way and will form a neuroma. A nerve graft is recommended for a gap of more than 2 cm in major peripheral nerves and more than 1 cm in digital nerves (Irwin, 1999). A clean, highly vascular recipient bed is necessary for nerve grafting (Irwin, 1999) and the graft should not be placed under tension. Tonkin (1997) noted that there was little evidence that vascularized grafts were better than non-vascularized grafts unless the recipient bed was avascular.

Nerve transfer

Tonkin (1997) suggested the use of nerve transfers following brachial plexus lesions, when a nerve root avulsion occurs and a nerve graft is inappropriate. However, Tonkin (1997) also highlighted the resultant problems in loss of function from the donor nerve's target organs. The aim of the nerve transfer is to restore motor function by inserting motor innervation near to the target muscle (Nath and Mackinnon, 1999).

Neurolysis

This technique consists of freeing the nerves from any adherent scar tissue to facilitate gliding.

Tendon repair

Primary repair: direct suture of lacerated tendons is most effective if done acutely, that is, before excessive retraction of the proximal portion of the tendon or the development of adhesions or joint stiffness.

A variety of suturing techniques can be utilized. The most common technique used to repair flexor tendon injuries is the Kessler or Modified Kessler suture. This involves a locking suture that approximates the two tendon ends, then an epitendinous circumferential suture that smoothes the surface of the repair to prevent snagging on the sheath and pulleys during tendon gliding (Figure 4.13). However, there are numerous methods of tendon repair, including grasping, non-grasping and multistrand techniques (Winters et al., 1997).

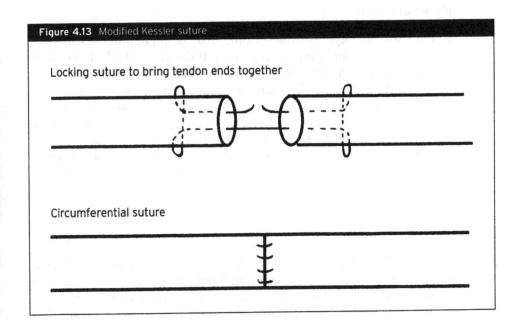

Figure 4.13 Modified Kessler suture

Locking suture to bring tendon ends together

Circumferential suture

If the flexor digitorum profundus (FDP) tendon has been divided close to its insertion (less than 1.5 cm), the proximal stump may need to be sutured directly to the distal phalanx. To secure the repair the sutures are brought through the digit and out via the nail, where a button is attached (*see* Figure 4.14). This button must remain in place for 6 weeks.

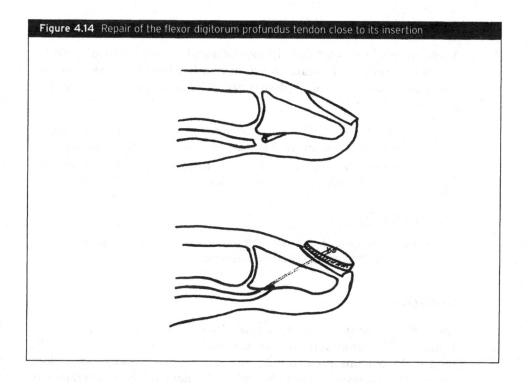

Figure 4.14 Repair of the flexor digitorum profundus tendon close to its insertion

Secondary repair: primary tendon suture may not be possible because of poor condition of the tendon ends or loss of the tendon. If a repair of these types of injury was attempted it could result in a tight repair, leading to loss of joint range of motion, or re-rupture of the tendon. In this situation a two-stage tendon reconstruction is necessary. First, a silicone rod is inserted into the flexor sheath to maintain its patency, then 3 months later, when the tissues have recovered from the initial trauma; the rod is removed and replaced with either a tendon transfer or graft. During the period that the rod is *in situ* the patient must maintain full passive flexion of the digit to prevent joint stiffness.

Tendon graft

A less vital tendon can be harvested and utilized to reconstruct a missing tendon. The plantaris and the palmaris longus are commonly used in this way (Harvey Kemble and Lamb, 1984). The proximal end of the tendon is sutured to the remaining stump of the original tendon and the graft is then tunnelled through the tissues and secured to the insertion by suturing it to the bone or the remnant tendon stump.

Tendon transfer

A tendon may be divided from its insertion and transferred to an alternate insertion in order to recreate an action that has been lost owing to neurological damage or tendon destruction. Common examples of tendon transfers in the hand are:

- the transfer of extensor indicis to the distal stump of a ruptured extensor pollicis longus tendon, when primary repair of this tendon is not possible
- the transfer of flexor carpi radialis to extensor digitorum to restore finger extension following a radial nerve injury.

Further reading

- Boscheinen-Morrin J, Conolly WB (2001) The Hand: Fundamentals of Therapy. Oxford: Butterworth-Heinemann.

Tenolysis

This refers to the freeing of a tendon from adhesions that are preventing it gliding. This procedure may be necessary after tendon repairs in the hand if the tendons become adherent to the flexor sheath, bone, skin, nerves, etc. Tenolysis is only indicated if all other conservative treatments have failed to free the adhesions and if the patient is willing to co-operate with the intensive post-operative exercise regime that is necessary to prevent reformation of adhesions (Boscheinen-Morrin and Conolly, 2001). Cannon (1989) reported that the aim of tenolysis of the flexor tendons within the hand was to restore intra-operative passive tendon motion so that active muscle contraction would result in an improved tendon glide and therefore a greater ranger of digit motion.

Indications for tenolysis include:

- a passive range of motion greater than the active range
- anticipated improvement in hand function
- motivated and compliant patient
- soft, supple tissues Cannon (1989).

Toe-to-hand transfer

To reconstruct a missing digit, a toe can be transferred to the hand. Most commonly, the second toe is used to replace a lost finger, but harvesting of the great toe is also possible, particularly when reconstructing a lost thumb. The aim of surgery is to provide a sensate digit and to restore a functional pinch grip (Bucchieri et al., 2002). In addition to this, a toe-to-hand transfer should provide digit length, a degree of motion and acceptable cosmesis.

Replantation

(*See* Chapter 10, case study 5.)

References

Anthony MS (1997) Skin grafts and flaps. In: GL Clark, EF Shaw Wilgis, B Aiello, D Eckhaus, L Valdata Eddington Hand Rehabilitation, A Practical Guide (second edition). London: Churchill Livingstone.

Bailie F (1997) Early wound excision and grafting. In: C Bosworth Burns Trauma: Management and Nursing Care. London: Baillière Tindall.

Bonavita L (1985) Free tissue transfer. American Journal of Nursing 885: 384-7.

Boscheinen-Morrin J, Connolly WB (2001) The Hand: Fundamentals of Therapy. Oxford: Butterworth-Heinemann.

Brcic A (1990) Primary tangential excision for hand burns. Hand Clinics 6: 211-19.

Bucchieri J, Poole BT, Schmidt CC, Baratz ME (2002) Restoration of thumb function after partial or total amputation. In: EJ Mackin, AD Callahan, TM Skirven, LH Schneider, AL Osterman Rehabilitation of the Hand and Upper Extremity (fifth edition). St Louis, MI: Mosby.

Buntic RF, Buncke HJ (1999) Principles of microvascular free tissue transfer. In: J Weinzweig J Plastic Surgery Secrets. Philadelphia, PA: Hanley & Belfus, chapter 83.

Cannon NM (1989) Enhancing flexor tendon glide through tenolysis and hand therapy. Journal of Hand Therapy Apr–Jun: 122-37.

Cason JS (1981) Treatment of Burns. London: Chapman & Hall.

Coull A, Wylie K (1990) Regular monitoring: the way to ensure flap healing. Nursing priorities following flap repair and reconstruction surgery. Professional Nurse October: 18-21.

Daane SP (1999) Leeches. In: J Weinzweig Plastic Surgery Secrets. Philadelphia, PA: Hanley & Belfus, chapter 85.

Davies D (1996) Principles of skin cover. In: RM Kirk, AO Mansfield, J Cochrane Clinical Surgery in General (second edition). London: Churchill Livingstone.

Edwards K (1994) Skin flaps in plastic surgery: an overview. Nursing Standard 9: 27-30.

Harvey Kemble JV, Lamb BE (1984) Plastic Surgical and Burns Nursing. London: Baillière Tindall.

Heimbach D, Luterman A, Burke J, Cram A, Herndon D, Hunt J et al. (1988) Artificial dermis for major burns: a multi-centre randomized clinical trial. Annals of Surgery 208: 313-20.

Irwin MS (1999) Nerve repair and regeneration. British Journal of Hand Therapy 4: 8-12.

Kim JH, Kim KC (1999) Principles of skin grafts. In: J Weinzweig Plastic Surgery Secrets. Philadelphia: Hanley & Belfus, chapter 79.

Leveridge A (1991) Therapy for the Burn Patient. London: Chapman & Hall.

Mankani MH, Pribaz JJ (1999) Free flap donor sites. In: J Weinzweig Plastic Surgery Secrets. Philadelphia, PA: Hanley & Belfus, chapter 84.

McGregor AD, McGregor IA (2000) Fundamental Techniques of Plastic Surgery and their Surgical Applications (tenth edition). London: Churchill Livingstone.

Munster AM, Weiner SH, Spence RJ (1990) Cultured epidermis for the coverage of massive burn wounds, a single centre experience. Annals of Surgery 211: 676-79.

Nath RK, Mackinnon SE (1999) Peripheral nerve injuries. In: J Weinzweig Plastic Surgery Secrets. Philadelphia: Hanley & Belfus, chapter 102.

Quaba A (1995) Reconstructive ladder for skin and soft tissue defects. Surgery: 126-32.

Ranelli S, Forsythe S, Nanchahal J (2000) Principles of rehabilitation in reconstructive surgery in the upper limb. British Journal of Hand Therapy 5: 5-9.

Reus WF, Colen LB, Straker DJ (1992) Tobacco smoking and complications in elective microsurgery. Plastic and Reconstructive Surgery 89: 490-3.

Roehr SP, Khan U, Healy CMJ (1997) Scars and scar revision. British Journal of Hand Therapy 2: 4-8.

Settle JAD (1996) Principles and Practice of Burns Management. London: Churchill Livingstone.

Sheridan RL, Hegarty M, Tompkins RG, Burke JF (1994) Artificial skin in massive burns – results to ten years. European Journal of Plastic Surgery 17: 91-3.

Singer DI, Moore JH, Byron PM (1995) Management of skin grafts and flaps. In: JM Hunter, EJ Mackin, AD Callahan Rehabilitation of the Hand: Surgery and Therapy. St Louis, MI: Mosby.

Soutar DS, McGregor IA (1986) The radial forearm flap in intraoral reconstruction: the experience of sixty consecutive cases. Plastic and Reconstructive Surgery 78: 1-18.

Stotland MA, Kerrigan CL (1999) Principles of skin flap surgery. In: J Weinzweig Plastic Surgery Secrets. Philadeliphia, PA: Hanley & Belfus, chapter 80.

Tompkins RG, Burke JF (1996) Alternative wound coverings. In: DN Herndon Total Burn Care. London: WB Saunders.

Tonkin MA (1997) Brachial plexus surgery. British Journal of Hand Therapy 2: 4-9.

Valauri FA (1991) The use of medicinal leeches in microsurgery. Blood Coagulation and Fibrinolysis 2: 185-7.

van Adrichem LAN, Hovius SER, van Strik R, van der Meulen JC (1992) The acute effect of cigarette smoking on the microcirculation of a replanted digit. Journal of Hand Surgery 17A: 230-4.

Weinzweig N, Weinzweig J (1999) Soft tissue coverage of the hand. In: J Weinzweig Plastic Surgery Secrets. Philadelphia, PA: Hanley & Belfus.

Winters SC, Seiler JG, Woo SL, Gelberman RH (1997) Suture methods for flexor tendon repair. A biomechanical analysis during the first six weeks following repair. Annales de Chirurgie de la Main 16: 229-34.

Chapter 5

The multidisciplinary team

Introduction

As with all specialities within healthcare, a team approach is essential to providing an optimal service to patients and their carers. In recent years, the definition of roles within the team has become increasingly blurred, with nurses, occupational therapists and physiotherapists extending their roles. Often, this blurring of definitions is caused by financial pressures on the NHS, as well as the personal career development of healthcare professionals. It is an opportunity for healthcare workers to continue to develop their careers from their previous highest grades without having to go exclusively into managerial work. This situation offers great benefits to patients as well as clinicians as their experience and knowledge is not lost. However, these new role definitions need clarifying in order to to avoid confusion and the replication of services (Biggs et al., 1998).

As with any effective team, the members need to work together and to respect each others' expertise and opinions (Pessina and Ellis, 1997). Teams do require leadership, but this role can be interchangeable in different situations. For example, case conferences are often led by consultants, who use the expertise of other team members to establish the facts of the medical case and to develop a treatment plan. However, therapists who wish to develop a rehabilitation or discharge plan, but who need input from other members of the multidisciplinary team, may initiate and lead a case conference.

The development of a team relies upon personalities: a very strong character who is unwilling to listen to others' opinions will limit the effectiveness of a team. Similarly, a very underconfident team member, who finds it difficult to express opinions, could also limit the team's progress. Essentially, the keystone to an effective and efficient team is communication and respect (Biggs et al., 1998).

The roles of a number of team members are discussed in this chapter. The list is not exhaustive, but it will introduce the professionals encountered most often. It may not be necessary for all members of a team to be involved with every patient, but this is how the dynamics of a good team should work, so that each team member knows their role and those of the others, and can provide their aspect of the service as needed. Team members should all complement each other to provide an optimal service to patients and their carers.

Further reading

Demling RH (1995) The 1995 presidential address: the advantage of the burn team approach. Journal of Burn Care and Rehabilitation 16(6): 569-72.

Key point

Communicate to achieve an effective multidisciplinary team that provides optimal patient care.

Patients

The purpose of the team is to provide the best possible care for patients. However, it should not be forgotten that patients and their carers are an integral part of the team and should be treated as such. Their opinions and wishes should be taken into consideration and they need to be involved in the decision-making processes. If patients and carers are involved in this way, and are made to feel involved in their own treatment, they will be more compliant with their rehabilitation (Groth and Wulf, 1995). This will help them to gain independence and take responsibility for their lives sooner, aiding earlier discharge and easier reintegration into society.

Relatives or friends

Families and friends also need to be involved in patients' treatment. After severe trauma they will need an immense amount of support and explanation from the medical team, but eventually – as they understand the treatment process – they can provide continuity of care and reinforce what the team is trying to achieve.

Surgeons

Patients' care is co-ordinated by the medical team throughout their treatment, from the time of admission to outpatient clinical reviews. Initially, surgeons are responsible for assessing patients' injuries and obtaining wound coverage by whichever plastic surgical techniques are most appropriate (see Chapter 4). After burn injuries, treatment most commonly involves debridement of necrotic tissue and split skin grafting (see Chapter 4). Once patients have recovered from the initial trauma of their injury, and wound coverage has been achieved, surgeons monitor them and may be required to perform further reconstructive procedures, for example to release skin contractures, to improve the cosmetic results of scarring and to free structures from adhesions.

In the case of elective surgery, surgeons are responsible for discussing surgical options with patients, and deciding with patients which procedure is the most appropriate for them as individuals. Many patients have unrealistic expectations about what plastic surgery can do for them, and fully discussing options with them and giving careful explanations of the likely outcome can achieve informed consent to surgery.

Anaesthetists

Patients may require multiple anaesthetics for surgical procedures and dressing changes; these, and management of patients' analgesia, are the responsibility of anaesthetists along with the rest of the medical team.

Nurses

Nurses have an ideal opportunity to monitor patients, to assess and reassess their condition, to identify patients' needs and to facilitate timely interventions, because of their continuous patient contact. Nurses develop a close rapport with patients and their families, and from this are able to provide psychological support and explanations of treatment. The need for this relationship is even more evident when nurses are caring for injured children and their parents. Nurses become patients' advocates but also have an important role in education as the principles of plastic surgery reconstruction can be difficult to understand (Edwards, 1994).

Because of their close contact with patients, nurses are often the first to identify patients' needs, for example analgesia requirements or loss of functional ability. It is then the responsibility of nurses to inform the appropriate members of the team to arrange specific treatments. Nurses are also responsible for administering prescribed treatments. This not only involves the administration of medications but also maintaining positioning or splintage and continual reinforcing of functional activity.

Burns and plastic surgery nurses are experts in wound management: this involves the use of appropriate wound assessment tools, cleansing agents and dressings to achieve optimum conditions for tissue healing. Even once wound closure has been achieved, the nursing staff will be able to educate patients about aftercare for the future.

The progression and familiarity of plastic surgery means that the relatively simpler surgical techniques, such as skin grafts and minor flaps, are now more commonly encountered on general surgical and orthopaedic wards (Edwards, 1994). This is a potentially controversial issue as nursing staff (and the rest of the team) caring for these patients may not be familiar with their specific requirements. One solution to this problem is the development of outreach services from the plastic surgery unit to provide advice, support and training to the various specialities.

Physiotherapists

Physiotherapists are vital in the rehabilitation of hand-injured patients (see chapters 6, 7 and 9), and any patient undergoing plastic surgery. However, for rehabilitation to be effective other team members should reinforce the treatment prescribed by physiotherapists. For example, if the physiotherapist is encouraging a patient to use the hand after reconstructive surgery, it is essential that nursing staff are aware of this requirement and also encourage function by allowing the patient to feed themselves, etc., rather than giving assistance. Nursing staff, physiotherapists and occupational therapists need to work together, with good communication, to ensure that everyone works towards agreed goals (Biggs et al., 1998).

The ultimate objective of rehabilitation is for patients to return to full independence, managing their former occupation and hobbies wherever possible (Harden and Luster, 1991). To achieve this physiotherapists must be involved in patients' care from day one (Fletchall and Hickerson, 1997) and everyone, including patients, must have a clear understanding of the aims of physiotherapy (Clarke, 1997).

The aims of physiotherapy in hand trauma and plastic surgery are to:

- educate
- maintain joint and soft tissue extensibility

- control oedema
- maintain or restore muscle strength or endurance
- re-educate sensation
- aid functional independence
- provide psychological support.

The treatment modalities used by physiotherapists to achieve these aims are many and varied (*see* Chapter 9).

Occupational therapists

During patients' hospital admissions occupational therapists are involved in the re-education of functional activities (both personal and domestic); this involvement may include visits to patients' homes and assessment of any aids that may be needed to facilitate independence. Occupational therapists also play an important role in the reintegration of patients back into society and to the workplace by providing opportunities to mix with other patients in group work and by dealing with concerns about work retraining and hardening.

However, the modification of scar tissue is the area in which the expertise of burns and plastic surgery occupational therapists is essential. Occupational therapists will assess, monitor and treat scars. The aims of occupational therapy for hand trauma patients are to:

- educate
- maximize function
- strengthen
- improve cosmesis
- minimize psychological dysfunction.

The treatment modalities that are most commonly used by occupational therapists are:

- education and support
- scar massage
- pressure garments
- silicone
- exercise
- splintage
- functional re-education.

Further reading

Gollup R (2002) Burns aftercare and scar management. In Bosworth Bousfield C (Ed) Burns Trauma, Management and Nursing Care. London: Whurr Publishers.
McGourty LK, Givens A, Fader PB (1986) Roles and functions of occupational therapy in burn care delivery. Journal of Burn Care and Rehabilitation 7(5): 431-3.

Dieticians

Although not usually necessary for patients with isolated hand trauma, the advice of a dietician is essential for patients who have pre-existing dietary problems or after more extensive trauma, for example large burn injuries. Injury creates a huge metabolic demand on the body, which if not anticipated and treated appropriately, can cause weight loss and delay tissue healing (Norman, 1997). Dieticians assess patients' nutritional needs and monitor their fulfilment closely. Factors that may affect the nutritional requirements of individual patients are:

- the extent of injury, that is, the size and depth of the burn
- age
- weight
- surgical, nursing and paramedical procedures
- sepsis
- pain
- pre-existing medical disorders
- nutritional status before injury.

During the rehabilitative phase, dieticians may need to adjust patients' nutritional intake to allow them to exercise optimally and to build muscle strength and exercise tolerance (Demling and DeSanti, 1998).

Further reading

Norman L (2002) Nutritional care for an individual following burn trauma. In: Bosworth Bousfield C (Ed). Burns Trauma, Management and Nursing Care. London: Whurr Publishers.

Social workers

Many patients require assistance from social workers. They may need any amount of help, for example advice about financial assistance that they can claim whilst they are recovering from their injury.

Psychologists

Any injury can be devastating and patients, along with their carers, may require support to come to terms with the trauma. Patients who need elective reconstructive surgery may also require psychological support. After the trauma, continued support will be needed as patients move on from the initial shock to the realization of the implications of their injury on their future lives, from living with resulting scars to altered family dynamics. The early involvement of a psychologist can assist patients to come to terms with their injury or surgery, to deal with any flashbacks and post-traumatic stress, and to re-adjust to society. All burns and plastic surgery units should have a psychologist working on their team. However, Van Loey et al. (2001) demonstrated that there was a need to improve psychological aftercare provided to burns patients, and Taal and Faber (1998) found that 33% of burn-injured patients still exhibited severe post-traumatic stress symptoms. All members of the multidisciplinary team should be involved in supporting patients and their carers. This was demonstrated by Rivlin et al. (1986), who showed that a decrease in parental anxiety could be achieved when a multidisciplinary approach to counselling was instituted.

Further reading

Bousfield C (2002) Psychological care following burn trauma. In: Bosworth Bousfield C (Ed) Burns Trauma, Management and Nursing Care. London: Whurr Publishers.
Antebi D (1993) The psychiatrist on the burns unit. Burns 19(1): 43-6.
Gilboa D, Shafir R, Tsur H, Floro S (1984) A team work model in a burns unit with the integration of a clinical psychologist. Burns, Including Thermal Injury 10(3): 210-13.

Prosthetists

Despite advances in reconstructive surgery there are still limitations to what plastic surgeons can achieve. The role of prosthetists is to provide patients with prostheses that are cosmetically acceptable. Prostheses are becoming more advanced with the developments of new materials and skills of prosthetists. They are usually either secured mechanically or are adhesive. However, it is even possible for surgeons to insert metal clips into patients, onto which prostheses can be clipped. Silicone implants that will fill depressions beneath pressure garments may also be needed. Jones (1997) reported that the cosmesis of hands is important because of the extent that they are involved in social contact and expression via gesticulation. The most common hand prostheses are the single-sleeve digit to replace an amputated digit or part of digit. These are made of silicone with an acrylic nail. These single digits may aid the resolution of oedema and facilitate some functional activities, such as keyboard skills, but they can inhibit range of joint motion and limit sensory input.

Cosmetic camouflage nurses

Scarring is inevitable after any injury or surgery. Scars can be treated and modified to achieve the best results possible, but they are still there and are usually visible. Cosmetic camouflage nurses are skilled in the application of cosmetic products that cover and mask scars, and it is their role to teach patients how to apply these products so that they can use them as they feel necessary. The best results are obtained when covering flat scars; raised or depressed scarring cannot be covered so well. The cosmetics are available on NHS prescription and this treatment can benefit men, women and children by increasing their confidence.

Further reading

Allsworth J (1985) Skin Camouflage: a Guide to Remedial Techniques. Cheltenham: Stanley Thornes.

Nursery nurses or play therapists

To treat children effectively takes time and patience. Staff must develop a relationship with them so that they are trusted despite the fact that what they are doing could be causing discomfort. With the limitations of funding and resources within the NHS, many rehabilitative staff simply do not have the time to spend developing these links with children and their carers, making co-operation with the treatments that they need difficult. The development of the role of play therapist and the nursery nurse can solve this problem. These members of the team have the experience of working with and caring for children so that by working alongside therapy staff they may be able to achieve the desired results. A physiotherapist who sees a child for a half-hour treatment session is less likely to be able to convince them to use an injured hand than the nursery nurse who is caring for and playing with the child all day. If the physiotherapist can liaise with the nursery nurse, explaining what movements are required, for example, the nursery nurse can incorporate this into a game or include an exercise session when the child is more co-operative.

Self-help groups

The development of self-help or survivor groups is becoming more commonplace. These groups are often connected with the regional burns unit and are supported by the staff, but are run by patients and their families. It is sometimes useful for members of these groups who have learnt to come to terms with their injuries to come to talk to new patients, as they are the only ones who really know exactly how it feels to sustain such an injury and to undergo surgery and rehabilitation.

Photographers

With advancement of technology, the way that patients are referred to the regional burns and plastic surgery unit is altering. It is now possible to take digital images in Accident and Emergency departments, which can then be sent for review and advice on treatment by the burns and plastic surgery unit medical and nursing staff via a computer link (Telemedicine). Patients therefore receive the most appropriate treatment and decisions can be made as to whether transfer to the specialist unit is necessary.

During treatment, medical photographers are involved in recording injuries and their progress. This is particularly useful for teaching purposes and these photographs are more commonly being used in accident litigation.

An excellent development is the use of digital photography in theatre during surgery. Images can then be reproduced on operation notes kept in patients' medical notes, and are therefore available for examination by the rest of the team. In this way, the other members of the team can fully understand the operative procedure.

Because of the nature of burns and plastic surgery services in the UK, many patients are transferred to outlying treatment areas that are closer to their homes after their discharge from the regional unit. The therapists and nursing staff in these areas may see burns and plastic surgery patients infrequently and be unfamiliar with appropriate treatments. Gallagher et al. (1990) suggested the use of visual documentation of wounds/rehabilitation regimes by use of videotaping.

References

Biggs KS, de Linde L, Banaszwski M, Heinrich JJ (1998) Determining the current roles of physical and occupational therapists in burns care. Journal of Burns Care and Rehabilitation 19(5): 442-9.

Clarke J (1997) Burns to the hands – the perspective from Roehampton. British Journal of Hand Therapy 2(6): 9-10.

Demling RH, DeSanti L (1998) Increased protein intake during the recovery phase after severe burns increases the body weight gain and muscle function. Journal of Burn Care and Rehabilitation 19(2): 161-8.

Edwards K (1994) Skin flaps in plastic surgery: an overview. Nursing Standard 9(4): 27-30.

Fletchall S, Hickerson WL (1997) Managed health care: therapist responsibilities. Journal of Burn Care and Rehabilitation 18(1): 61-3.

Gallagher J, Lakatos M, Goldfarb IW, Slater H (1990) Discharge videotaping: a means of augmenting occupational and physical therapy. Journal of Burns Care and Rehabilitation 11(5): 470-1.

Groth GN, Wulf MB (1995) Compliance with hand rehabilitation. Journal of Hand Therapy 8(1): 18-21.

Harden NG, Luster SH (1991) Rehabilitation considerations in the care of the acute burn patient. Critical Care Nursing Clinics of North America 3(2): 245-53.

Jones S (1997) The prosthetists role in partial finger loss. British Journal of Hand Therapy 2(7): 20-1.

Norman L (1997) Nutritional care in burns patients. In: Bosworth C (Ed) Burns Trauma, Management and Nursing Care. London: Baillière Tindall.

Pessina MA, Ellis SM (1997) Burn management. Rehabilitation. Nursing Clinics of North America 32(2): 365-74.

Rivlin E, Forshaw A, Polowyj G, Woodruff B (1986) A multidisciplinary group approach to counselling the parents of burned children. Burns, Including Thermal Injuries 12(7): 479-83.

Taal LA, Faber AW (1998) Post-traumatic stress and maladjustment among adult burn survivors 1-2 years post-burn. Burns 24(4): 285-92.

Van Loey NE, Faber AW, Taal LA (2001) Do burns patients need burn specific multidisciplinary outpatient aftercare: research results. Burns 27(2): 103-10.

Part 2

Role of the physiotherapist

Chapter 6

The role of physiotherapists in the care of the burned hand

Introduction

Physiotherapists are vital in the rehabilitation of burn-injured patients. However, a team approach to patient care is essential (*see* Chapter 5), and the roles of individual members of the multidisciplinary team often overlap (Biggs et al., 1998). Nursing staff, physiotherapists and occupational therapists all need to work closely together to ensure that everyone works towards agreed goals (Biggs et al., 1998). The ultimate objective of rehabilitation is for patients to return to full independence, managing their former occupations and hobbies wherever possible (Harden and Luster, 1991). To achieve this, everyone, including patients, must have a clear understanding of the aims of physiotherapy (Clarke, 1997).

Hand burns require physiotherapy from the earliest stage of wound management (Kealey and Jensen, 1988). Finger and thumb joints are very sensitive and range of motion can be lost quickly. The burned hand becomes grossly oedematous, and uncontrolled oedema collects on the dorsum of the hand where the tissues are loose. This causes the metacarpophalangeal joints to hyperextend, stretching the long flexor tendons of the hand so that the interphalangeal joints are pulled into flexion; the result is a clawed hand. In this position the joint structures (ligaments and volar plates) are in their shortened position and will contract, rendering the hand useless (*see* Chapter 7). It is therefore imperative that the hand is kept elevated in a Bradford sling at all times to allow the oedema to drain (Figure 6.1).

Aims of physiotherapy

- To prevent joint contracture.
- To aid functional independence.
- To provide psychological support.

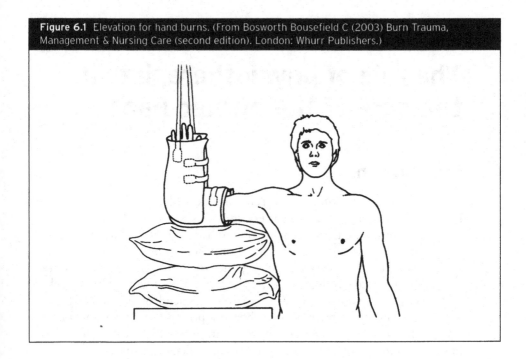

Figure 6.1 Elevation for hand burns. (From Bosworth Bousefield C (2003) Burn Trauma, Management & Nursing Care (second edition). London: Whurr Publishers.)

Prevention of joint contracture

It is important to differentiate between a skin contracture and a joint contracture. Damaged or grafted skin contracts as it heals (*see* Chapter 1). If this skin covers a joint, the joint will be pulled into the direction of the contracture. If identified early enough a release of the skin contracture will allow resumption of full joint range of motion. However, if the skin contracture is allowed to persist the joint structures that are being held in a shortened position, such as ligament, capsule, volar plate or muscle, will also contract. Joint structures, and hence a joint contracture, are extremely difficult to release surgically and their rehabilitation is lengthy, therefore joint contractures must be prevented (Boswick, 1983) and early physiotherapy intervention that aims to do this can delay or alleviate the need for later surgical reconstruction (Bahnof, 2000).

Key point

During treatment sessions physiotherapists must take great care not to contaminate patients' wounds. Meticulous hand washing before and after treatment, plus the use of gloves and an apron, provide the best means of preventing infection.

Exercise

Regular exercise of affected joints is encouraged as soon as possible after patients are admitted. Exercise not only maintains joint range of motion but also aids oedema drainage by producing a muscle pump (Grigsgy de Linde and Miles, 1995). Total active and passive ranges of motion are monitored and patients are taught exercises (*see* Chapter 9) to obtain isolated tendon gliding and intrinsic muscle activity (Grigsgy de Linde and Miles, 1995).

Dressings should be as light as possible so that patients can exercise regularly, both under the supervision of the physiotherapist and independently. The use of plastic or semi-permeable membrane bags are ideal as they allow free movement of the digits (Gairns and Martin, 1990; Martin et al., 1990). Physiotherapists encourage patients to move each affected joint through as full a range of movement as possible (Kealey and Jensen, 1988). If this cannot be achieved physiotherapists use passive exercises (Grigsgy de Linde and Miles, 1995).

An ideal time for physiotherapists to encourage patients to exercise is during bathing (Raeside, 1992). Dressings do not impede movement and it is often more comfortable for patients to move in warm water. Treatment sessions in this instance are kept brief to avoid patients getting cold. Pain control is essential (Raeside, 1992) and physiotherapists should endeavour to time exercises with the administration of analgesia. If oral analgesia is not effective, and circumstances permit, physiotherapists can administer Entonox (*see* Chapter 9) during treatments (Roe and Peck, 1999).

Care should be taken when treating patients with burns to the dorsum of the hand as the extensor tendons, particularly the central slip of extensor digitorum tendon, over the proximal interphalangeal joint can easily be exposed. Rupture of the central slip results in a Boutonnière deformity of the finger. Sheridan et al. (1995) identified that only 9% of patients who sustained damage to the extensor mechanism of their hand achieved normal function.

Exercise is stopped for 5–7 days after skin grafting to allow the grafts to heal (Carmudie, 1980; Clarke, 1997). However, more recently it is the author's experience that this timescale is being further reduced to 3 days. Once the skin grafts are stable, exercise can be resumed. Initially, this should be with the dressings off so that the grafts can be observed (Grigsgy de Linde and Miles, 1995).

Exercise becomes a regular part of patients' daily routine and to facilitate this, physiotherapists, along with the rest of the team, should encourage them to achieve their dietary requirements in order to maintain energy levels. Physiotherapists encourage, advise and progress the exercise programme, but responsibility for exercise is gradually given to patients. This responsibility for rehabilitation is the start of patients' progression towards independence.

Initially, the aim of exercise is to maintain full joint range of motion. Eventually, physiotherapists alter the emphasis of the programme towards regaining muscle strength, motor control, endurance and function.

Most young children do not require physiotherapy treatment as they do not lose joint range of motion as quickly as adults (Clarke, 1997). If exercise is necessary, physiotherapists need to use their imagination when devising play activities to encourage movement at the required joints (Raeside, 1992). The assistance of the nursery nurse can be of great benefit in these circumstances (*see* Chapter 5).

The use of continuous passive motion machines in the rehabilitation of hand injuries is increasing (Adams and Thompson, 1996). Salter (1996) advocated their use and demonstrated a reduction in pain, maintenance of range of motion, reduction in complications and a shorter period of rehabilitation. However, Pope et al. (1997) investigated their use after surgery to the lower limb and demonstrated no significant improvement in function or range of motion. Of greater concern is the identification of increased blood loss and analgesic requirement (Pope et al., 1997). However, the application of repeated sub-maximal stress to scar tissue has been shown to be effective in achieving tissue lengthening (Kisner and Colby, 1990).

Positioning

The position the patient rests and sleeps in needs to be monitored to control oedema and prevent contractures (Boswick, 1983). Most frequently, the position of comfort is that of flexion. However, if a patient is permitted to rest in this position constantly the joints will begin to contract. (*See* Chapter 7 for position of safe immobilization.)

Splinting

(*See also* Chapter 9.) Patients who are fully compliant with exercise or who are minimally burned do not require splintage (Richard et al., 1996). However, if exercise and positioning are not sufficient in maintaining correct alignment of a joint, a splint is required (Schnebly et al., 1989). Initially, splints are worn at all times, only being removed for change of dressings and twice daily by physiotherapists so that full range of active or passive movements can be carried out. The physiotherapist or occupational therapist will usually make the splint from thermoplastic material that is heated in hot water to soften it (Carmudie, 1980). When sufficiently cool the splint is moulded over the patient's dressings to hold the joint in the corrected position. The splint material becomes virtually rigid once it is completely cool. The splint is secured by a bandage or Velcro straps (Figure 6.2 and Figure 6.3). Eventually, splints may only need to be worn at night, leaving patients free to use the injured part and exercise regularly during the day.

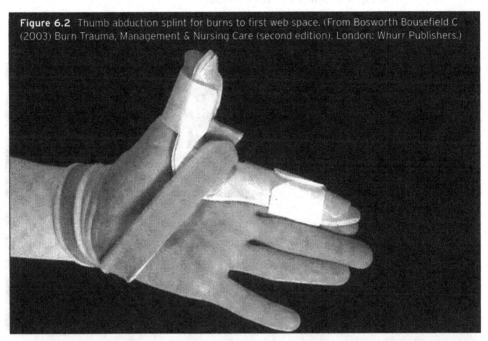

Figure 6.2 Thumb abduction splint for burns to first web space. (From Bosworth Bousefield C (2003) Burn Trauma, Management & Nursing Care (second edition). London: Whurr Publishers.)

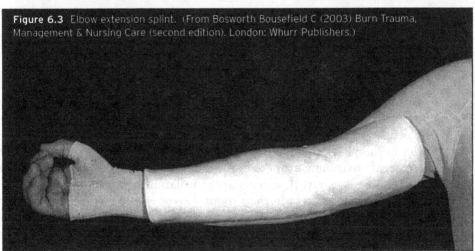

Figure 6.3 Elbow extension splint. (From Bosworth Bousefield C (2003) Burn Trauma, Management & Nursing Care (second edition). London: Whurr Publishers.)

Splinting is particularly important for patients with hand burns who are ventilated and sedated and are therefore unable to co-operate with exercises. The hands are splinted in a position that will prevent joint contractures (Figure 6.4):

- *wrist*: 15-30° of extension
- *metacarpophalangeal joints*: 45-80° of flexion
- *interphalangeal joints*: full extension
- *thumb*: abduction and 10-20° of flexion at metacarpophalangeal joint and extension at interphalangeal joint (Bach et al., 1984).

Figure 6.4 Hand resting splint. (From Bosworth Bousefield C (2003) Burn Trauma, Management & Nursing Care (second edition). London: Whurr Publishers.)

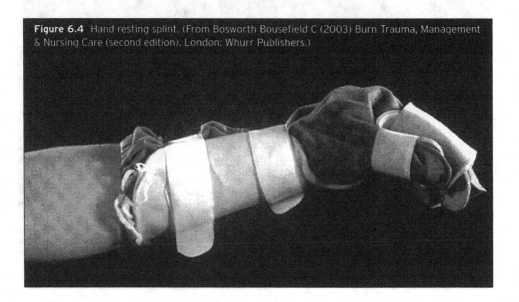

Aid functional independence

Strengthening

Muscle strength, exercise tolerance and endurance are developed by gradually increasing the frequency and intensity of exercise sessions (Hartigan et al., 1989). Patients are encouraged to make use of the facilities in the physiotherapy department gym. This removes them from the protected environment of the burns unit and begins their preparation for the return to society. If patients are in isolation because of wound infection, equipment is kept in their room. Parrot et al. (1988) demonstrated that although a structured exercise circuit for burn-injured patients resulted in no change in the length of hospitalization, it did reduce the number of outpatient therapy visits required. Ideally, after discharge from hospital there should be the facility for patients to attend outpatient rehabilitation regularly, in order to gradually increase their muscle strength and endurance.

Self-care and independence

As preparation for discharge home, patients are encouraged to be independent in all daily activities (Giuliani and Perry, 1985). Patients with injured hands should use them for functional activities as well as continuing with regular exercise. They need to be as independent as possible, particularly if they live alone.

Physiotherapists need to work closely with patients and other members of staff to achieve these goals. It may be necessary for physiotherapists to visit patients' homes to assess their individual needs.

Psychological support

Most burn-injured patients have difficulty in coming to terms with their injuries and go through various stages of anxiety, depression or even aggression (Giuliani and Perry, 1985). Physiotherapists have an ideal opportunity to establish relationships with patients during treatment sessions, and are able to offer support and encouragement when necessary. The parents of burned children may need to supervise exercises or appropriate play activities when their child returns home (Raeside, 1992). Parents need help and support at this time, particularly if their child is unwilling to co-operate. Patients often have many questions and anxieties about scarring, altered body image and how they will manage at home or work. These anxieties may be voiced to physiotherapists during treatment sessions and, when appropriate, physiotherapists are able to offer reassurance and advice.

Key point

Patients who are encouraged to assume responsibility for their rehabilitation will achieve a greater sense of motivation and accomplishment (Gripp et al., 1995).

Outpatient follow-up

After discharge from the burns unit, hand burns need to be monitored for some time to ensure that any graft tightness does not result in joint contracture, so patients may need to continue with physiotherapy treatment as outpatients (Raeside, 1992). Physiotherapists normally review patients when they attend for a change of dressing, as this makes it is easier to monitor joint movement.

Van Loey et al. (2001) demonstrated that a quarter of burns patients were dissatisfied with exclusively medical doctor follow-up clinics, and suggested that there may be a need for multidisciplinary outpatient clinics.

Conclusion

Patients' functional outcome is dependent on an integrated team approach at all stages of their recovery (Clarke, 1997). Physiotherapists have an important and often demanding role in the rehabilitation of burn-injured patients, requiring patience, adaptability and often a firm but caring approach. The ability to work with other members of the multi-disciplinary team is essential as it is close teamwork that will help patients to overcome their injuries. Each patient requires individual assessment and re-assessments, a prescriptive regime is inappropriate (Clarke, 1997) except during the initial management of mass casualty incidents (Barillo et al., 1997).

Further reading

Leveridge A (1991) Therapy for the Burn Patient. London: Chapman & Hall.
Chartered Society of Physiotherapy and College of Occupational Therapy (2000) Standards for Burns. London: Chartered Society of Physiotherapy.

References

Adams KM, Thompson ST (1996) Continuous passive motion use in hand therapy. Hand Clinics 12(1): 109-27.
Bach J, Draslov B, Jorgensen B (1984) Positioning, splinting and pressure management of the burned hand. Scandinavian Journal of Plastic and Reconstructive Surgery 18: 145-7.
Bahnof R (2000) Intra-oral burns: rehabilitation of severe restriction of mouth opening. Physiotherapy 86(5): 263-6.
Barillo DJ, Harvey KD, Hobbs CL, Mozingo DW, Cioffi WG, Pruitt BA (1997) Prospective outcome analysis of a protocol for the surgical and rehabilitative management of burns to the hands. Plastic and Reconstructive Surgery 100(6): 1442-51.
Biggs KS, de Linde L, Banaszewski M, Heinrich JJ (1998) Determining the current roles of physical and occupational therapists in burn care. Journal of Burn Care and Rehabilitation 19(5): 442-9.

Boswick JA (1983) Rehabilitation after burn injury. Annals of the Academy of Medicine 12(3): 443-8.

Carmudie C (1980) Management of the burned hand. Australian Journal of Physiotherapy 26: 4.

Clarke J (1997) Burns to the hands - the perspective from Roehampton. British Journal of Hand Therapy 2(6): 9-10.

Gairns CE, Martin DL (1990) The use of semi-permeable membrane bags as hand burn dressings. Physiotherapy 76(6): 351-2.

Giuliani CA, Perry GA (1985) Factors to consider in rehabilitation aspect of burn care. Physical Therapy 66(5): 619-23.

Grigsgy de Linde L, Miles WK (1995) Remodelling of scar tissue in the burned hand. In: JM Hunter, EJ Mackin, AD Callahan. Rehabilitation of the Hand: Surgery and Therapy. London: Mosby.

Gripp CL, Salvaggio J, Fratianne RB (1995) Use of burn intensive care unit gymnasium as an adjunct to therapy. Journal of Burn Care and Rehabilitation 16: 160-1.

Harden NG, Luster SH (1991) Rehabilitation considerations in the care of the acute burn patient. Critical Care Nursing Clinics of North America 3(2): 245-53.

Hartigan C, Persing JA, Williamson SC, Morgan RF, Muir A, Edlich RF (1989) An overview of muscle strengthening. Journal of Burn Care and Rehabilitation 10(3): 251-7.

Kealey GP, Jensen KT (1988) Aggressive approach to physical therapy management of the burned hand. Physical Therapy 68(5): 683-5.

Kisner C, Colby LA (1990) Therapeutic Exercise, Foundation and Techniques (second edition). Philadelphia, PA: FA Davis.

Martin DL, French G, Theakstone J (1990) The use of semi-permeable membranes for wound management. British Journal of Plastic Surgery 43: 55-60.

Parrot, M, Ryan R, Parks DH, Wainwright DJ (1988) Structured exercise circuit program for burn patients. Journal of Burn Care and Rehabilitation 9(6): 666-8.

Pope RO, Corcoran S, McCaul K, Howie DW (1997) Continuous passive motion after primary total knee arthroplasty. Does it offer any benefits? Journal of Bone and Joint Surgery 79(6): 914-17.

Raeside F (1992) Physiotherapy management of burned children: a pilot study. Physiotherapy 78(12): 891-5.

Richard R, Staley M, Miller S, Warden G (1996) To splint or not to splint - past philosophy and present practice: Part 1. Journal of Burn Care and Rehabilitation 17(5): 444-53.

Roe A, Peck F (1999) Entonox - an effective analgesic for painful physiotherapy procedures. British Journal of Hand Therapy 4(2): 60-3.

Salter RB (1996) History of rest and motion and the scientific basis for early continuous passive motion. Hand Clinics 12(1): 1-11.

Schnebly WA, Ward RS, Warden GD, Saffle JR (1989) A non-splinting approach to the care of the thermally injured patient. Journal of Burn Care and Rehabilitation 10: 263-6.

Sheridan RL, Hurley J, Smith MA, Ryan CM, Bondoc CC, Quinby WC, Tompkins RG, Burke JF (1995) The acutely burned hand: management and outcome based on a ten year experience with 1047 acute hand burns. Journal of Trauma 38(3): 406-11.

Van Loey NE, Faber AW, Taal LA (2001) Do burns patients need burn specific multidisciplinary outpatient aftercare: research results. Burns 27(2): 103-10.

Chapter 7

Principles of hand therapy

Introduction

The hand is a multifaceted tool, therefore it is not surprising that treating its dysfunctions is a complicated and often daunting topic. The hand has an enormous capacity for motion and yet its opportunity for injury and disease, plus its psychological value, makes the restoration of dexterity and function one of the greatest challenges in physiotherapy.

Rest or mobilize?

There has been debate over whether to rest or mobilize injuries (Salter, 1996). Recently, early motion has been strongly advocated but it is important to recognize the stages of wound healing (*see* Chapter 1) and to arrange a balance between rest and exercise. For example, overaggressive manipulation of a joint during the inflammatory stage can prolong this phase and delay healing, but gentle stress during the fibroplastic phase assists the development of new collagen, and therapeutic stretching realigns collagen during scar maturation.

With the introduction of more aggressive treatment regimes for hand-injured patients the prognosis for many injuries that were once considered disastrous to hand function, is more positive. These regimes focus on earlier intervention to avoid the complications of interstructural adhesions and to promote resolution of oedema and tensile strength within the tissues. It has been demonstrated that these proactive regimes can work (Cullen et al., 1989) but this philosophy should not be taken too far.

Rest is an integral part of the delicate process of tissue healing (*see* Chapter 1). Effective healing relies upon a balance of rest and mobility (Ranelli et al., 2000), and the time that is allowed for rest should not be taken away by more and more 'early active regimes'. When considering the body's reaction to injury, the need for rest is demonstrated. During the phase of inflammation, the tissues swell and become painful. These reactions prevent movement and as physiotherapists, we should respect this stage of healing.

Gradually the swelling and pain subside and the patient is more willing to move. This change occurs as the body's healing process moves from inflammation to fibroplasia (*see* Chapter 1). Movement is necessary to encourage the rebuilding phase of the healing process, and this is the physiotherapists' optimal time of effect. They can work with patients to encourage the resolution of motion and function as the body rebuilds the structures within.

Key point

Therapeutic intervention is dependent upon, and should be tailored to, the stage of tissue healing.

The position of safe immobilization

The position that a patient's hand will adopt after injury is the position that the hand is at risk of contracting into, that is, a clawed hand (Figure 7.1). The position of safe immobilization (POSI) for the hand is the virtual opposite of this (Figure 7.2).

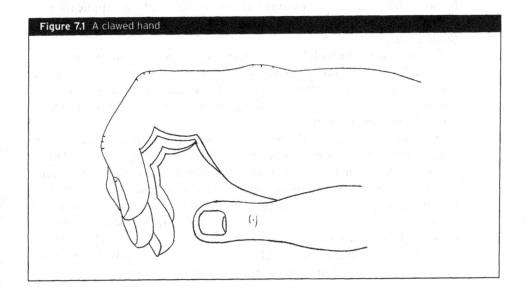

Figure 7.1 A clawed hand

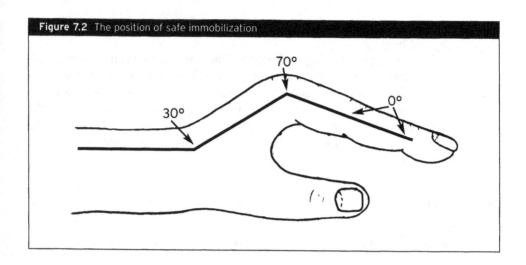

Figure 7.2 The position of safe immobilization

If necessary, the hand can be maintained in the position of safe immobilization by the use of a static splint (Figure 7.3). The principles of the position of safe immobilization are relevant to all types of hand positioning and splinting. The resting splint is the most commonly used static hand splint, and it incorporates all the optimal joint positions to prevent contractures. It is the position from which all other static splints are developed. Alterations to the position of safe immobilization are only necessary to remove unwanted stress from structures and to allow controlled exercise. For example, the wrist position is altered to neutral or slight flexion after repair of an extrinsic flexor tendon with the application of the splint to the dorsal aspect rather than the volar aspect of the hand (Figure 7.4).

The reason for immobilizing the hand in the position of safe immobilization is to maintain the joint structures in their taut or lengthened position. The aim is to prevent these joint structures from shortening during the inflammatory phase of healing, and to promote the resumption of full motion after its resolution.

If an injured hand is allowed to rest in an uncontrolled position the posture that it will adopt is that of a claw hand (*see* Figure 7.1). This is caused by the accumulation of oedema on the dorsal aspect of the hand, where the overlying soft tissues are more elastic and allow expansion (Collings, 1999) compared with the thicker palmar aspect. The skin over the dorsum of the hand stretches to accommodate the oedema and the resultant increased pressure alters the transverse and longitudinal arches of the hand (Sorenson, 1989). The soft tissue stretch pulls the metacarpophalangeal joints into hyperextension; in turn, this applies a stretch to

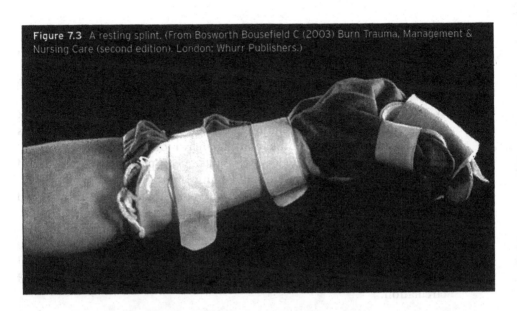

Figure 7.3 A resting splint. (From Bosworth Bousefield C (2003) Burn Trauma, Management & Nursing Care (second edition). London: Whurr Publishers.)

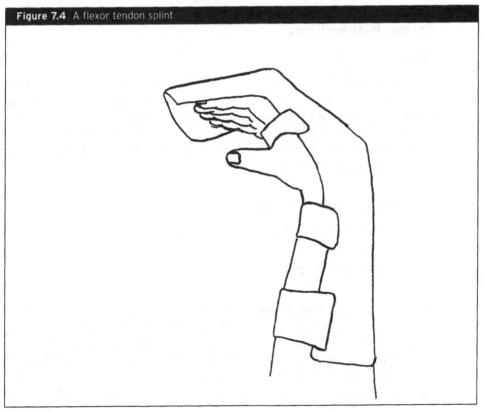

Figure 7.4 A flexor tendon splint

the extrinsic flexor tendons, and the interphalangeal joints are held in flexion. The intrinsic muscles of the hand are at mechanical disadvantage, preventing them from flexing the metacarpophalangeal joints and extending the interphalangeal joints (Collings, 1999). Oedema in the digit web spaces also causes the digits to abduct. The loss of soft tissue extensibility maintains the thumb in a position of metacarpophalangeal joint extension and adduction resulting in tightness of the flexor pollicis longus tendon, causing flexion of the interphalangeal joint.

Eventually, if this hand posture is allowed to persist, the excess fluid and exudate within the tissues will begin to fibrose, and if not opposed, the result will be loss of tissue glide and extensibility, joint stiffness and contractures leading to a reduction in hand function (Sorenson, 1989).

Kottke et al. (1966) demonstrated that immobilization caused connective tissue to contract, reorganize and become dense, subsequently restricting motion. This occurred within a week of immobilizing normal tissue but was magnified by the presence of oedema, trauma and impaired circulation.

Optimal joint positions

Wrist

The wrist should be positioned at 15–30° of extension to prevent flexion contracture. The wrist is vulnerable to flexion contracture because of the effects of gravity and the muscle imbalance of a greater number of flexors acting upon the joint than extensors. In addition, the maintenance of wrist extension will facilitate grip in the later stages of rehabilitation and the resumption of hand function.

Metacarpophalangeal joints

Diathroidal joints allowing three planes of movement:

- flexion-extension
- abduction-adduction
- rotation.

The metacarpophalangeal joints are unstable and rely on the collateral ligaments to secure their position. The collateral ligaments are loose in extension, thus allowing greater abduction and adduction in this position, and facilitating dexterity. When immobilizing the metacarpophalangeal joints they must be held in sufficient flexion to keep the collateral ligaments taut. The minimum amount of flexion needed is 40° with 80° being the comfortable maximum. This position will maintain the intrinsic plus posture of the hand and will support the transverse arch, preventing ligamentous damage.

Interphalangeal joints

Hinge joints allow flexion and extension only. They are stable and are supported by collateral ligaments. The ligaments are not at as much risk of shortening as those of the metacarpophalangeal joints, but the volar plate and the flexor sheath become compressed during joint flexion and will contract in this position. The extensor mechanism is also vulnerable as it splits into the central slip and lateral bands in this region. If the proximal interphalangeal joint is immobilized in flexion the central slip is at risk of rupture, causing unopposed flexion at the proximal interphalangeal joint and hyperextension at the distal interphalangeal joint (Boutonnière deformity). To protect against this and to maintain the length of the volar plates the interphalangeal joints are splinted in full extension, avoiding hyperextension.

Thumb

The ideal position of immobilization for the thumb is mid-opposition, slight flexion of the metacarpophalangeal joint and extension of the interphalangeal joint. This aims to maintain the first web space and prevent contracture. The first metacarpophalangeal joint differs to those in the fingers, it is flatter therefore allowing less movement, and the ligaments are less prone to damage.

Metacarpal arch

The splint must be moulded up into the metacarpal arch to prevent damage to the metacarpophalangeal joint volar plates and palmar subluxation of the joints. This may be difficult to achieve if oedema is extensive (Collings, 1999).

Principles of physiotherapy for hand injuries

The aims of physiotherapy intervention for a patient with any type of hand injury or surgery are to:

- promote patients' understanding of their injury or condition
- promote wound healing and manage resultant scarring

- control oedema
- manage pain
- maintain joint range of movement
- promote soft tissue extensibility
- aid recovery of sensibility
- restore muscle power
- restore function
- provide psychological support.

The treatment modalities used to achieve the above are discussed in Chapter 9. Not all patients will require all the above interventions, and the injury or surgery will determine which treatment modality takes priority.

Oedema

Oedema is worthy of specific analysis as, despite being needed for tissue healing, it causes the majority of complications after hand trauma and surgery.

The identification of the type and cause of oedema will assist the development of a treatment plan to alleviate it (Palmada et al., 1999). Sorenson (1989) noted that the maintenance of fluid balance in normal tissue relies upon a balance between the vascular and lymphatic systems.

Vascular system

The diffusion of fluid between the vascular system (that is, the capillaries) and the tissues is dependent upon the following.

- *Permeability of the capillary walls to water and proteins*: water passes freely out of the capillaries, but proteins are retained.

- *Hydrostatic pressure within the capillaries*: the higher the pressure, the more water is forced out of the vascular system and into the tissues.

- *Osmotic pressure*: the higher the concentration of proteins in the blood plasma, the greater the attraction of water; therefore, if the plasma protein concentration is raised, water is absorbed back into the capillaries from the tissues.

Lymphatic system

The lymphatic system drains interstitial fluid and plasma protein fractions back into the vascular system.

If the balance between the vascular system and the tissues is disrupted because of trauma, an excessive amount of fluid collects in the tissues and the mechanisms for its return to the bloodstream are either overwhelmed or destroyed. Excessive interstitial oedema results in loss of motion in the hand; however, the increased tissue pressure also causes ischaemia and will therefore either extend tissue damage or delay healing (Salter and Bexon, 2000).

References

Collings J (1999) The role of the fifth metacarpophalangeal joint in the recovery of the burnt hand - is it great or small? British Journal of Hand Therapy 4(1): 33-8.

Cullen KW, Tolhurst P, Lang D, Page RE (1989) Flexor tendon repair in zone 2 followed by controlled active mobilization. Journal of Hand Surgery 14B: 392-5.

Kottke FJ, Pauley DL, Ptak RA (1966) The rationale for prolonged stretching for correction of shortening connective tissue. Archives of Physical and Medical Rehabilitation 47: 345-52.

Palmada M, Shah S, O'Hare K (1999) Hand oedema: pathophysiology and treatment. British Journal of Hand Therapy 4(1): 26-32.

Ranelli S, Forsythe S, Nanchahal J (2000) Principles of rehabilitation in reconstructive surgery in the upper limb. British Journal of Hand Therapy 5(1): 5-9.

Salter RB (1996) History of rest and motion and the scientific basis for early continuous passive motion. Hand Clinics 12(1): 1-11.

Salter M, Bexon C (2000) Treatment. In: M Salter, L Cheshire (2000) Hand Therapy: Principles and Practice. Oxford: Butterworth-Heinemann.

Sorenson MK (1989) The edematous hand. Physical Therapy 69(12): 1059-64.

Chapter 8

Assessment of the hand

Introduction

Assessment is the foundation of our clinical practice. It is used to evaluate patients' baselines, their progress and the outcome of treatment. The use of appropriate assessment tools enables clinicians to select treatment techniques and then to measure their effectiveness.

Ideally, assessment techniques ought to have been proved to be valid and reliable. However, many of the tools that are commonly used for assessment, for example observational assessments, have no such evidence of their accuracy but are still valuable in the clinical setting, if not in research.

Key point

Data collection must be:

- interpretable
- accurate and repeatable
- valid
- standardized.

Reliability

The assessment method should provide consistent results on every occasion it is used and for every clinician that uses it. Below are listed some of the terms used to describe the different aspects of the reliability of an assessment:

- *Test-retest reliability*: the same result should be obtained on different occasions.
- *Inter-rater reliability*: the same result should be obtained by two or more assessors when evaluating the same patient.
- *Intra-rater reliability*: the same result should be obtained by the same assessor on the same subject on two or more occasions

(Bowling, 1997).

Validity

The assessment method that is chosen should be appropriate to obtain the information that is needed (Bowling, 1997).

Standardization

All clinicians should be able to conduct the assessment technique in the same way, with the same equipment.

Prerequisites to assessment

The solid foundation to any assessment is clinicians' knowledge of normal anatomy, physiology and biomechanics. It is the responsibility of clinicians to ensure that this knowledge is maintained and updated as necessary.

> Diagnosis is only a matter of applying one's anatomy (Cyriax, 1982)

History-taking and interviewing skills are sometimes underestimated. The most important aid to a diagnosis is the description given by the patient (Lamb, 1987), and it takes experience for clinicians to be able to draw out clear and concise histories from patients.

A sequential approach to the assessment is necessary to ensure that nothing is omitted. However, it is inappropriate to simply apply all known tests to patients, instruments must be selected for their appropriateness and developed as the assessment progresses.

Accurate documentation will allow comparison of findings at subsequent assessments. Knowledgeable interpretation of findings and progression of assessment will aid clinicians to move from assessment, to diagnosis and finally to goal-setting and treatment-planning.

Ellis and Bruton (1998) listed the main aims of assessment as:

- establishing a baseline measurement
- re-evaluation after intervention
- establishing an outcome measure
- a means of exchanging information
- evidence for research.

Assessment also motivates patients and may affect their compliance with their treatment programmes (Sorenson, 1989).

The following chapter lists the most common assessment methods and tools. This list is by no means all-inclusive and there are a number of specialized tests that could be added for particular conditions or injuries. However, the aim of the chapter is to provide a sound basis for assessment of the hand, and with experience, it is anticipated that readers' assessment techniques will expand and develop, in the same way as an assessment should progress, depending upon what is found. Inexperienced assessors will find it useful to have a pattern of assessment to follow, but as their confidence and experience grows, they will find that the results of one examination tool lead the direction of assessment. During assessment, it is appropriate to anticipate the irritability of the patient's condition and to alter the examination accordingly. It may be necessary to spread the assessment over a number of sessions to avoid increasing symptoms.

Subjective assessment

A thorough subjective assessment provides the solid foundations of an accurate objective assessment. Subjective questioning guides the progress of the objective examination. Clinicians begin to develop an idea of the possible diagnosis by appropriate questioning of patients, and this is explored further within the objective examination. Specific questions related to patients' general health are included to establish any pre-existing medical problems that may be affected by the examination and treatment. Whilst taking a subjective history, it is useful to observe the patient's affected hand for posture, resting position and level of use.

History of present condition

The following information should be noted:

- age and gender
- mechanism of injury or history of the condition, including dates
- progress since injury or surgery, or onset
- details and dates of surgical interventions
- behaviour of symptoms, that is, aggravating or easing factors
- hand dominance
- patients' evaluation of the main problem
- previous treatment and its effects.

Past medical history

Note the following information:

- systemic illness
- previous injury or surgery to the upper limb
- relevant previous injuries or surgery.

Drug history

This should include details of the following:

- medication(s) being used at present
- dosage of analgesia required
- known allergies to medications
- may include levels of smoking or alcohol consumption.

Social history

This should include details of the following:

- occupation
- hobbies
- social situation.

Objective assessment

Clinicians have a whole battery of examination techniques available to them in order to establish the causes of patients' symptoms. However, objective assessment does not simply involve performing a list of tests one after another. Clinicians must select the most appropriate tests for individual patients and develop them throughout the examination, interpreting their findings as the examination progresses.

For example, a patient may complain of reduced range of motion at the interphalangeal joint of the thumb. It is the physiotherapist's responsibility not simply to measure the loss of range of motion, but to establish the cause and implications of this loss of motion by examining:

- the muscles and tendons that produce the movement
- the peripheral nerves that elicit the movement
- the joint structures
- the level of comfort during the movement
- the functional limitations caused by the loss of motion.

This section is intended to demonstrate some of the most appropriate methods of examination. The most difficult part of assessment is interpreting the findings. A sound knowledge base of anatomy, physiology and the biomechanics of the structures of the upper limb is essential to enable clinicians to interpret findings and to understand how one anomaly will affect and interact with other structures.

Contents of an objective examination

The objective examination of patients should include the following:

- observation
- palpation
- soft tissues
- range of motion
- individual muscle tests
- grip strength
- sensation
- pain
- neurological function
- function
- specific tests
- psychological function.

If only one hand is affected, both should be compared in order to aid the identification of anomalies.

Observation

Note changes in the following:

- *Skin colour*: differences in skin colour suggest alterations in vascularity or conditions such as complex regional pain syndrome.
- *Nail changes*: any deformities should be documented.
- *Contour*: differences in contour are noted at this stage of the assessment, with a view to further investigation. Alterations in contour may be caused by oedema, deformity, muscle wasting or bony protuberances.
- *Oedema*: the site of swelling and its extent should be noted.
- *Wound*: the position of any wound is documented, as is the stage of healing and any signs of infection.
- *Scarring*: the stage of maturation, position and direction of scars is noted, for example, raised, red, linear scar over volar aspect of proximal inter-

phalangeal joint, right index finger. The presence of contractures is also noted.

- *Resting position and deformity:* the digits of the hand normally rest in a slightly flexed positioin, any alteration to this position in one or more digits should be obvious and indicates that further examination into the cause is needed. Common deformities, such as those caused by peripheral nerve palsies should be obvious and easily identified by clinicians.

At this stage it is also appropriate to examine any X-rays, scans or other reports from investigations.

Palpation

Note alterations in the following:

- *Skin temperature:* the temperature of the skin can be measured objectively by use of thermal electrodes. However, this practice is time-consuming and the equipment is rarely available in physiotherapy departments. Such accurate measures of skin temperature are only necessary in research situations. In practice, a simple comparison of the temperature between patients' affected and unaffected hands is adequate. Any alteration in temperature is most easily assessed by the examiner touching patients' hands with the dorsum of their hands (Bell-Krotoski et al., 1995). Alterations in temperature may signify circulatory anomalies or infection.
- *Contour:* alterations in contour that were identified in the initial observation of the hand can now be explored further to identify their cause, for example a prominence over the distal interphalangeal joint may be identified as an osteophyte, suggesting the presence of osteoarthritis.
- *Oedema:* on palpation it is noted whether the oedema feels soft or thickened. If chronic oedema has begun the process of fibrosis, indentations are left when the swelling is pressed firmly, this is documented as 'pitting oedema'.
- *Scar tissue:* it is noted whether scar tissue feels soft and pliable or is hard and tight.
- *Pain:* if the patient identifies any specific areas of the hand that are tender, painful or hypersensitive during palpation the anatomic site is noted and the cause of the discomfort investigated further.
- *Soft tissues:* palpation of the soft tissues of the hand and forearm will aid identification of areas of interstructural adherence.
- *Bones and joints:* palpation of joint lines and joint structures reveal anomalies that have not been identified visually.

Soft tissues

Oedema

Numerous factors affect oedema within the soft tissues:

- extent of soft tissue injury
- limb position
- time of day
- temperature – intrinsic and extrinsic
- level of recent activity
- recent treatment modality.

As far as is possible, the assessment of oedema should be carried out at the same time of day and after the same level of activity or treatment (Salter 1987; Sorenson, 1989).

Methods of assessment include the following:

- *Observation*: compare hands; note the extent of any oedema.
- *Palpation*: note the density of oedema.
- *Tape measure*: make a circumferential measurement; ensure accurate repeatability by noting the exact position of the measurement (Sorenson, 1989); a small weight can be attached to the end of the tape measure to ensure consistent application of tension in subsequent tests (Ewing Fess, 1995).
- *Ring measure*: graded rings that fit over a digit are used, and accuracy is improved if they are available in whole and half sizes.
- *Callipers*: external callipers are used to assess the diameter of localized swellings (Ewing-Fess, 1995).
- *Volumetric displacement*: a volumeter is filled with water to a measured level and the hand is immersed to a standardized level. The displaced water is collected and measured; this volume of displaced water can be compared at subsequent assessments. However, to ensure the reliability of this assessment a number of variables need to be considered. First, the measurement of the displaced water needs to be entirely accurate (Boland and Adams, 1996), as does the level to which the hand is immersed into the water (Bell-Krotoski et al., 1995). The temperature of the water (King, 1993) and the anatomical positioning of the hand (Bell-Krotoski et al., 1995) should be consistent in all assessments. Both Nicholas (1977) and Vasiliauskas et al. (1995) noted that hand dominance can also affect the size of the hand and therefore this should be allowed for when comparing hands. Cederlund (1998) concluded that the assessment of oedema by use of a volumeter could also be used to determine tissue response to intervention.

Scar tissue

The assessment of scar tissue can be limited to subjective description.

However, there are methods of examining scars more objectively, as follows:

- *Observation*: colour indicates level of maturity; breakdown indicates fragility; extent; hypertrophic - raised, red, confined to area of injury; keloid - raised, extends beyond area of injury; direction indicates potential for contracture.
- *Palpation*: texture; density; fragility; elasticity; tenderness; blanching; interstructural adhesions.
- *Measurement*: joint range of motion; elevation of scar tissue.
- *Dental impressions*: taking a 'dental impression' produces a three-dimensional model of the scar, but is a time-consuming and often clinically inappropriate technique (Sawada, 1994).
- *Photography*: made more accurate if a grid is added to the picture, but subsequent photographs need to be taken from identical positions and distances; expensive and time-consuming.
- *Vancouver scar scale*: Baryza and Baryza (1995) described a method of assessing all aspects of a scarring. The method is both reliable and objective (Grigsgy de Linde and Miles, 1995), and rates four characteristics of the scar tissue that relate to healing, scar maturity, cosmesis and function of healed skin. These characteristics are: pigmentation, vascularity, pliability and scar height.

Circulation
Methods of assessment of circulation include the following:

- *Colour*: a hand with compromised circulation appears pale or cyanotic; impaired venous drainage produces a dusky blue colour.
- *Pulses*: the radial and ulnar pulses may feel weak or be absent.
- *Capillary reflux*: skin colour blanches on compression and capillary reflux should be easily observed immediately after release; this may be slowed or absent if circulation is compromised.
- *Temperature*: skin temperature is directly related to vessel patency (Ewing Fess, 1995); normal digital temperature ranges between 30°C and 35°C (Ewing-Fess, 1995); assessment of differences in temperature is made by the examiner using the dorsum of the hand; more accurate measurements may be obtained by the application of cutaneous sensors, although this method is time-consuming and not relevant in clinical practice.
- *Doppler scan*: ultrasound is used to monitor arterial flow through audible responses to arterial pulsing; this technique is often used to assess vessel patency in donor sites before flap reconstruction.
- *Allen test* (Ashbell et al., 1967): this is a test for arterial patency first described by Allen in 1929; the examiner places the fingers over the

radial and ulnar arteries at the wrist; the patient forcibly opens and closes the hand to exsanguinate it, while the examiner occludes the arteries; the patient opens the hand and the examiner releases one artery then observes the flushing of the hand. If there is a reduction in blood flow through that artery this will be obvious by the lack of flushing; the Allen test can be used on individual digits by applying the compressive pressure over the digital arteries.

Skin and nails

The integrity and condition of the skin and nails of patients' hands is very informative. Diagnosis of conditions or injuries is aided, and evidence of disuse is apparent. The following methods of assessment may be used.

- *Observation*: alteration in colour may indicate vascular or neural changes, for example a disturbance in the autonomic supply to the hand.

- *Hydration*: the skin may appear dry or scaly, this could be caused by nerve injury or disuse.

- *Integrity*: thin, papery skin with bruising commonly occurs in patients with rheumatoid disorders. Denervated areas of skin are smooth and thin as epidermal atrophy leads to reduced dermal ridging. The pulps of the digits may also become atrophied and appear tapered making the whole digit appear smaller. The absence of calluses on the hands of a patient who has thickened skin and calluses on the uninjured hand is a sign of disuse, and persistent ulceration can be caused by loss of protective sensation, reduced vascularity, a retained foreign body, instability of scar tissue or factitious wounds (Callahan, 1995).

- *Wounds*: divided into superficial, partial and full thickness skin loss. Superficial wounds will appear red, will be very painful and will have a rapid capillary reflux. Partial thickness wounds will have a patchy red colour, may have blistered, have a reduced sensation and a slow capillary reflux. Full thickness wounds will appear white or black (depending upon the mode of injury) and may be pain-free because of the destruction of the nerve endings (Boscheinen-Morrin et al., 1992).

- *Hair*: denervation can cause hair to fall out or become longer and finer, increased hair growth is termed 'hypertrichosis'.

- *Cleanliness*: an excessively clean hand or part of hand, such as one digit, suggests that the patient is not using it functionally. An area that is denervated has decreased skin creases and sweating, therefore dirt retention is reduced.

- *Nails*: ridged and brittle nails occur after nerve injury. Nail spicules may persist if any of the germinal matrix remains after excision. Ganglions can produce longitudinal nail splitting and infections in the nail fold are common (paronychia).

On palpation:

- *Temperature: see* assessment of circulation.
- *Sweating:* the examiner is able to detect differences in sweating by simple palpation - tactile adherence test (*see* special tests).
- *Texture:* comparison of the integrity of the skin surface with other uninjured areas, and palpation of scar tissue and contractures will establish tight areas.
- *Elasticity:* areas of reduced elasticity will be apparent on palpation and passive movements.
- *Tenderness:* whilst palpating the skin areas of tenderness may become apparent.

Range of motion

The assessment of joint range of motion is used commonly by physiotherapists as it is often the most obvious of symptoms and is easily measured. However, methods of assessment vary greatly, as does the equipment that is used and the ways in which results are recorded. Clinicians must first identify why they are measuring joint range of motion.

Initially, loss of motion may be examined to establish a diagnosis, for example loss of active extension of the interphalangeal joint of the thumb is suggestive of a rupture of the extensor pollicis longus tendon. Once an accurate diagnosis has been made, the measure of joint range of motion is then used to evaluate effectiveness of treatment. Simple joint range of motion should not be used as a way of assessing hand function, as patients with severely limited movement are still able to use their hands adequately.

When assessing the range of motion of a joint, clinicians also assesses the quality of that motion. For example, the patient may be able to achieve full extension of all of the fingers but on examination it is noted that the proximal interphalangeal joint of the middle finger initially sticks in flexion, then achieves a sudden full range of extension on increased effort by the patient, this is suggestive of 'trigger finger'. If only range of motion is recorded, this vital piece of evidence would be missed and could lead to misdiagnosis.

The following types of joint motion require assessment:

- active
- passive
- accessory.

The choice of which type of joint motion is assessed depends on clinical reasoning and the pathology being evaluated (Ellis and Bruton, 1998). Clinicians should note the cause of any alteration in range of motion, for example 'patient complains of end of range stiffness or pain' or 'therapist feels a block to passive range of motion'. The ranges of joint movement are measured to establish a baseline of motion and to monitor alterations in motion and therefore assess the outcome of therapeutic intervention.

There are numerous methods available to assess range of motion of the hand. These include visual estimation of joint range, measurement of the distance between the finger-tip and the distal palmar creases, and mapping joint range by use of wires, tracing or shadows. However, although these methods of examination are relatively simple to apply, their reliability is questionable.

It has been demonstrated by Bruton et at. (1999) that ranges and standard deviations for visual estimation of joint ranges were considerably larger when compared with goniometry. This substantiates the findings of previous investigations (Hellibrant et al., 1949; Moore, 1949).

Measurement of the distance between finger tip and distal palmar crease only gives global measurement of all joint ranges (Boyes, 1950) rather than identification of individual joint range of motion, for example it is possible to touch the distal palmar crease with the finger tip whilst maintaining the metacarpophalangeal joints in extension, as in a hook fist. Therefore, repeated measures of joint range by use of this method would not identify any improvement or deterioration of range of metacarpophalangeal joint motion.

The advancement of technology will create more accurate methods of measuring joint range of motion. At present, developments include electric goniometers and the data glove (Ellis and Bruton, 1998).

Goniometry
The validity of goniometry depends on assessors' knowledge of anatomical landmarks and biomechanics. There has been an enormous amount of research into every aspect of the use and application of goniometry. Essentially, if used in a standardized manner, goniometry is a reliable and valid measure of joint range of motion (Goldsmith and Juzi, 1998). However, it has been demonstrated that a difference of more than 5° should only be accepted as significant between different assessors (Boone et al., 1978). Solgaard et al. (1986) noted that intra-rater reliability of goniometry is greater than inter-rater reliability, suggesting that differences in measurements of less than 5° can be accepted as significant when the same physiotherapist measures the same joint in the same way with the same equipment.

Despite goniometry being generally accepted as a reliable and effective assessment tool, it has been demonstrated by Pratt and Burr (2001) that there are still limitations to this method of evaluation. When examining the use of goniometry by hand physiotherapists in the British Isles, more than 19 styles and makes of goniometer were identified as being used, with only 41% of respondents reporting the use of a standardized protocol for their measurement techniques (Pratt and Burr, 2001).

When measuring joint range of motion the position of the surrounding joints is noted and standardized for subsequent measurements, that is, when measuring metacarpophalangeal joint flexion, the positions of the interphalangeal joints are noted. Starting positions of the hand need to be documented (Figure 8.1).

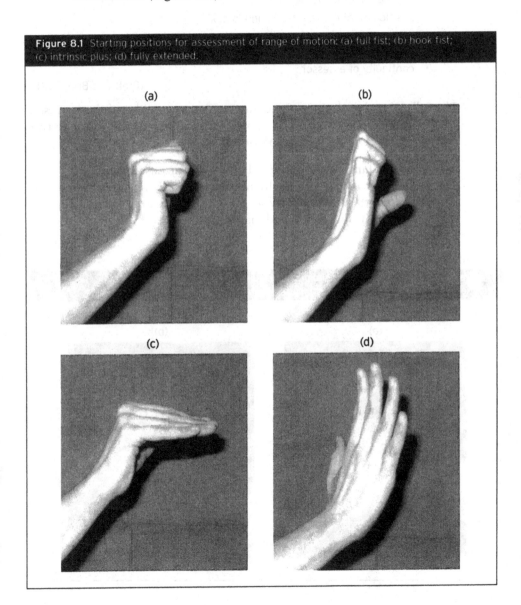

Figure 8.1 Starting positions for assessment of range of motion: (a) full fist; (b) hook fist; (c) intrinsic plus; (d) fully extended.

Placement of the goniometer also affects the reliability of the measurement and subsequent assessments (Pratt and Burr, 2001). Further research is needed into the application of goniometry in hand therapy, but until this is established the most accurate way of measuring joint range of motion is to set a standardized protocol for the following:

- type or make of goniometer used
- application of the goniometer
- position of joint and surrounding joints
- method of reading off results from the goniometer, for example to the nearest 5°
- continuity of assessor

(Pratt and Burr, 2001).

The following descriptions of measurement are examples of those chosen by the author as the easiest to apply and repeat, but are not definitive ways of measuring joint range of motion.

Metacarpophalangeal and interphalangeal joint measurement

The goniometer is placed dorsally over the joint. The patient is asked to flex or extend the joint actively as far as possible whilst verbal encouragement is given (Figure 8.2 and Figure 8.3).

Figure 8.2 Metacarpophalangeal and proximal interphalangeal joint measurement: (a) metacarpophalangeal range of motion; (b) proximal interphalangeal range of motion

(a)

(b)

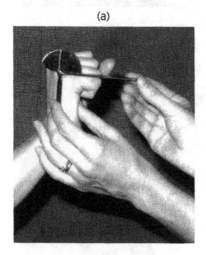
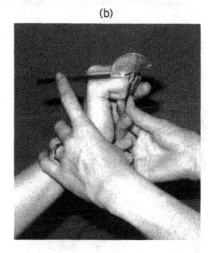

Figure 8.3 Distal interphalangeal and thumb interphalangeal joint measurement: (a) distal interphalangeal range of motion; (b) thumb interphalangeal range of motion

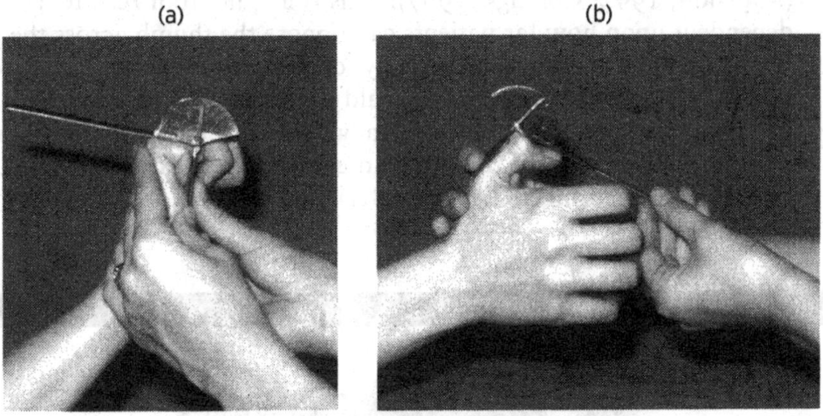

Total active motion (TAM) or total passive motion (TPM) is calculated by adding the sum of the measurements for extension of all the joints of one digit and subtracting this from the sum of the measurements for flexion of all the joints of the same digit. This reflects the general mobility of the hand (ASSH, 1976), but does not identify specific information about individual joints and therefore should not be used to reflect function (Ellis and Bruton, 1998).

Calculation of total active flexion (TAF)
TAF = metacarpophalangeal flexion + proximal interphalangeal flexion
      + distal interphalangeal flexion
Example:
        TAF = 90° + 100° + 60°
        TAF = 250°

Calculation of total lack of active extension (TLAE)
TLAE = metacarpophalangeal extension deficit + proximal interphalangeal extension
       deficit + distal interphalangeal extension deficit
Example:
        TLAE = 10° + 30° + 15°
        TLAE = 55°

Calculation of total active movement (TAM)
TAM = TAF − TLAE
Example:
        TAM = 250° − 55°
        TAM = 195°

First carpometacarpal joint measurement

A quick and useful method of measuring the range of motion at the carpometacarpal joint of the thumb is the use of the Kapandji scale (Kapandji, 1992; Collings, 1997). This is a scale from zero to 10 that is dependent upon how far patients can oppose the thumb across the palm. For example, if a patient can actively touch the thumb tip to the tip of the middle finger, the measurement would be noted as active range K4. If the clinician were able to increase this range passively to enable the thumb tip to approximate with the tip of the little finger, the measurement would be noted as passive range K6 (Figure 8.4).

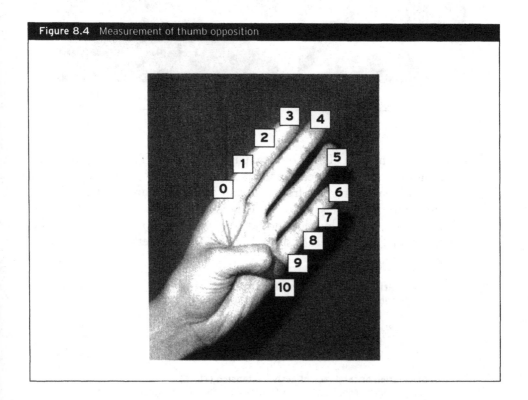

Figure 8.4 Measurement of thumb opposition

Radiocarpal joint measurement

When measuring flexion and extension at the wrist, patients are positioned with their elbows supported on the table and their forearms vertical. Measurements are taken along the ulnar border of the arm or hand and neutral is taken as 0° for both directions. The arms of the goniometer lie along the line of the ulna and the fifth metacarpal (Figure 8.5).

Figure 8.5 Radiocarpal joint flexion and extension measurement: (a) wrist flexion; (b) wrist extension

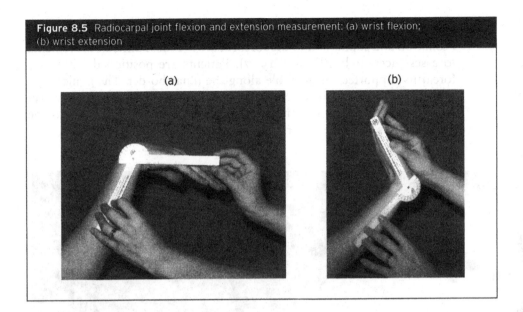

Radial and ulnar deviation at the wrist is measured by placing the hand palm-down on the table. The axis of the goniometer is placed over the joint and the distal arm is positioned along the middle finger, which is generally accepted to be the mid-position of the hand. Measurements are taken either side of this neutral position (Figure 8.6).

Figure 8.6 Radiocarpal joint radial and ulnar deviation measurement: (a) wrist radial deviation; (b) wrist ulnar deviation

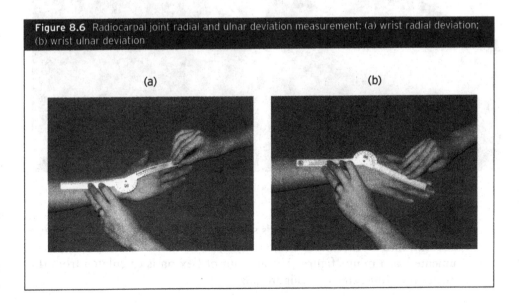

Superior radio-ulnar joint measurement

Pronation and supination of the forearm are the most difficult movements to assess accurately (Wagner, 1977). Patients are positioned with their forearms supported on the table along the ulnar border. The goniometer is held on one side of the forearm and patients are asked to rotate the arm away from it. One arm of the goniometer remains vertical, whereas the other follows the patient's arm (Figure 8.7).

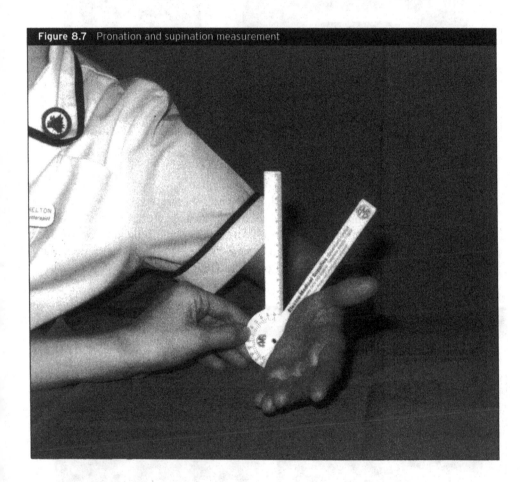

Figure 8.7 Pronation and supination measurement

Elbow joint measurement

The arm is placed by the patient's side with the forearm in a mid-position of rotation. Full extension is stated as 0°, and any loss of extension is documented as a minus figure. The amount of flexion is calculated from the position of full extension (Figure 8.8).

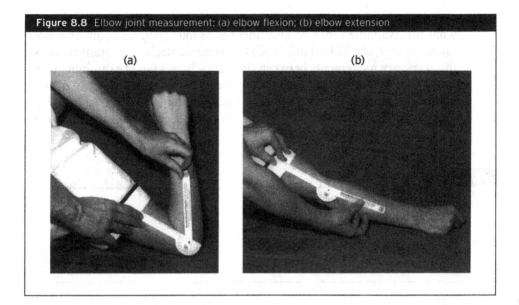

Figure 8.8 Elbow joint measurement: (a) elbow flexion; (b) elbow extension

(a)   (b)

Reasons for inaccuracies in measurements include the following:

- pathology, for example alterations in level of oedema between measurements; pathology affecting bony contours and joint alignment (Ellis and Bruton, 1998)
- inconsistent starting position
- inconsistent patient effort
- inexperience of assessor
- different assessors
- inconsistent placement of goniometer
- altered amount of force applied through goniometer arms
- inconsistency in documentation of results.

Passive physiological range of motion
The measurement of passive range of motion with goniometry is less reliable than the measurement of active range of motion because of the opportunity for varied pressures being applied to the arms of the goniometer (Ellis and Bruton, 1998).

Accessory range of motion
Accessory joint movements are the small gliding and rotational movements that occur within a joint during normal movement to facilitate the full range of motion, but which cannot be achieved in isolation, for example the rotation of the base of the proximal phalanx on the metacarpal head during the gripping of a spherical object. Accessory movements are

used to assess joint integrity. The direction of movement is noted, as is what the available range of movement feels like: stiff, lax, pain at end of range, absent, etc. (Maitland, 1992). It is particularly important to assess the accessory movements between the carpal bones when examining hand motion as alteration in the gliding between these bones can have a marked effect on the surrounding joints. Kaltenborn (1980) described 10 intercarpal or radiocarpal movements that are useful to ensure all aspects of the carpus are examined.

Key point

Assessment of motion includes
- active motion
- passive motion
- accessory motion

Individual muscle tests

The assessment of individual muscles and tendons gives information about their innervation and continuity. To assess the individual action of each of the muscles in the hand and forearm there is no substitute for accurate and extensive anatomical and biomechanical knowledge. With this sound foundation, any alterations to the normal are apparent, and it is then the responsibility of the clinician to examine the cause of the abnormality. This could be obvious, for example the absence of active extension of the metacarpophalangeal joint of the middle finger associated with a laceration over the dorsum of the wrist must indicate a division of the extensor digitorum tendon to the middle finger. However, it may be less clear, for example a suspected median nerve lesion demonstrating all the expected sensory and motor deficiencies except that the patient still has the ability to produce flexion at the metacarpophalangeal joint of the thumb. Anatomical knowledge will demonstrate that the ulnar nerve can innervate the deep head of flexor pollicis brevis.

The application of resistance to muscle groups and individual muscles will also provide information about the state of the tendons that convey motion. Resistance can be applied to produce either an isometric contraction of a muscle, or joint motion is allowed to produce an isotonic contraction.

A sound knowledge base of normal anatomy and biomechanics is an essential prerequisite to assessment and evaluation.

Grip strength

The terminology used to describe the different postures of grip varies widely. Figures 8.9, 8.10 and 8.11 demonstrate the terminology used at Nottingham City Hospital. Clinicians should be wary when comparing trial data from different studies, as it is essential to establish exactly which grips were measured.

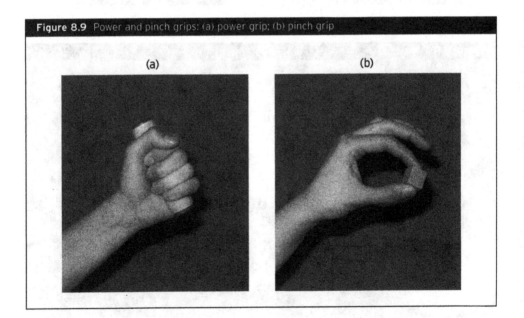

Figure 8.9 Power and pinch grips: (a) power grip; (b) pinch grip

(a)   (b)

Figure 8.10 Lateral pinch and hook grips: (a) lateral pinch grip; (b) hook grip

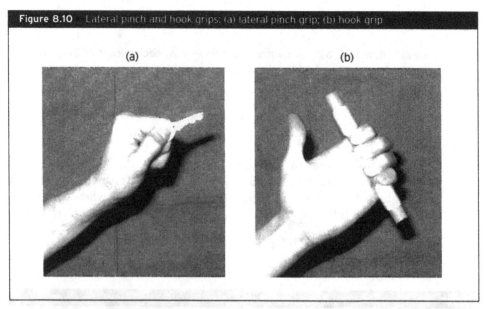

(a)   (b)

Figure 8.11 Tripod grip

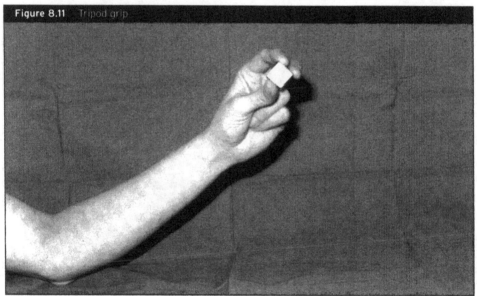

Factors affecting the assessment of grip strength include the following:

- *Hand dominance*: the dominant hand will be slightly stronger than the non-dominant hand.
- *Age*: strength diminishes with age, but this should not be assumed.

A comparison of hands gives physiotherapists an indication of patients' normal grip strength unless both hands are affected.

- *Pain*: if the patient is suffering discomfort during the examination of grip strength, the measurement may be reduced.
- *Sensation*: the brain relies on the sensory and proprioceptive information it receives to control the hand. If this information is lacking, patients may find function difficult, therefore creating disuse of the hand and subsequent atrophy of the musculatures.
- *Joint range of motion*: if joint motion is limited the muscles do not achieve their full excursion, if this persists they will atrophy. Also, if full range of motion is not achievable, patients may have difficulty using the grip-strength measuring device.
- *Hand size*: patients with small hands may have difficulty using certain grip-strength measurement devices.
- *Comprehension of instructions*: if patients do not understand how the measurement is to be made they may not be able to achieve maximal strength. This can be helped by ensuring that patients receive adequate instruction, demonstration and practice.
- *Psychological status*: it is difficult to assess patients' motivation to achieve a maximal grip strength measure and to identify low-effort patients. Stokes et al. (1995) described a model that can be used to categorize patients into those who are making little effort and those who are sincere. However, this method is time-consuming and requires specialist equipment.

Grip strength is usually tested using isometric muscle activity, for example by dynamometry. Isotonic assessment involves the movement of a weight through a range of motion and therefore numerous other variables will affect the result. Thus, work simulators such as the Baltimore Therapeutic Equipment (BTE) work simulator are ideal for this type of assessment.

Methods of assessment of grip strength include the following:

Oxford scale

This is a subjective measurement of muscle power in relation to gravity or resistance. However, varying starting positions or altering verbal commands can elicit different results. The scale is rated from zero to five: 0 = nothing; 1 = flicker of muscle contractility; 2 = complete range of motion with gravity eliminated; 3 = complete range of motion against gravity; 4 = complete range of motion against gravity and moderate resistance; 5 = normal.

Hand-held dynamometry

The hand-held dynamometer has been proved reliable when used in a standardized manner (Bechtol, 1954). It also has good inter-rater, intra-rater and test-retest reliability (Maithiowetz, 1991). However, assessment of pinch grip is less reliable as it is a finer action that requires stability of a series of joints.

There are published standardized protocols (Gilbertson and Barber-Lomtax, 1994) that state that the dynamometer should not be allowed to rest on the table for support but if the patient is unable to manage the weight of the equipment physiotherapists may give some assistance by holding the gauge (Figure 8.12). The optimal setting for maximal grip strength is level two (Firrell and Crain, 1996).

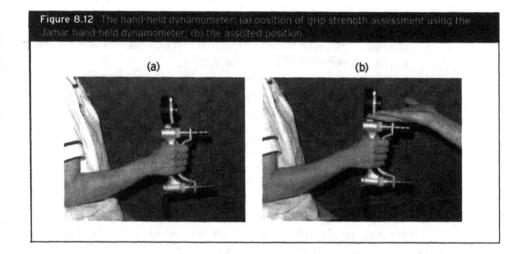

Figure 8.12 The hand-held dynamometer: (a) position of grip strength assessment using the Jamar hand-held dynamometer; (b) the assisted position

(a)   (b)

Grip strength is strongest with the forearm supinated and weakest in pronation (Richards et al., 1996). Ng and Fan (2001) demonstrated that the position of the elbow also affects grip strength when measured using a hand-held dynamometer. It was found that grip strength was significantly lower when the elbow was held at 120° flexion and that it was highest when the elbow was at 90°.

The hand-held dynamometer is also able to provide information about consistency of patient effort (Hildreth and Breidenbach, 1989), but the calibration of the equipment should be checked regularly to ensure consistency.

Figure 8.13 Assessment of pinch and lateral grips: (a) pinch grip position; (b) lateral pinch grip position

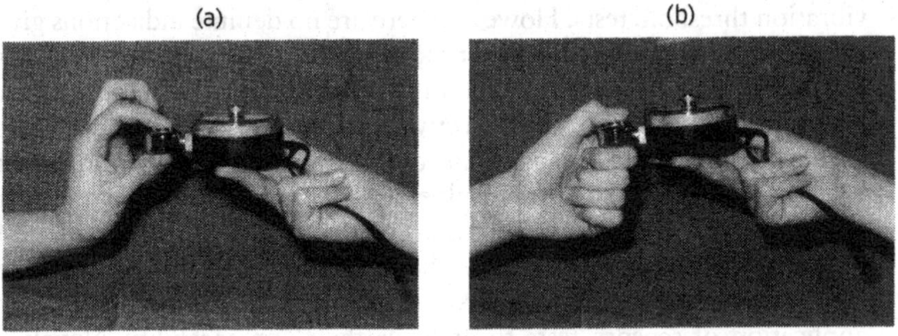

Sensation

Sensibility in the hand forms the basis for normal function. The information gained from sensory receptors facilitates skilful motor control of the hand. There are numerous sensory assessment techniques available to physiotherapists. These tests must be evaluated and compared to ensure that the most appropriate investigation method is used for individual patients. It is most appropriate that the methods of examination should all have a functional bias. If possible, the test should require the patient to manipulate an object rather than passively allow the examiner to perform the test. Callahan (1995) states that sensation is assessed more accurately if the patient's hand is allowed to actively explore an object, as this is how the hand works within its natural environment.

Callahan (1995) divided the available sensory assessment techniques into four categories:

- *Threshold tests*: these evaluate the minimum stimulus that patients can identify accurately, for example the monofilament test.
- *Functional tests*: these assess the quality of sensibility that is present within the hand, that is, whether patients' sensation is adequate for precise, discriminative function or simple, gross manipulation of objects, for example stereognosis.
- *Objective tests*: these do not correlate to hand function but are simply applied to patients in a standardized manner to achieve an objective measurement of nerve recovery, for example nerve conduction studies.
- *Stress tests*: these tests aim to provoke intermittent symptoms to facilitate diagnosis, for example the Phalen test.

Mielke et al. (1996) noted that four sensory tests dominated both the literature and clinical practice. These were: the static two-point discrimination; the dynamic two-point discrimination; the pressure threshold; and the vibration threshold tests. However, there are no definite indications given in the literature concerning appropriate selection of these techniques. Mielke et al. (1996) noted that some studies that aimed to evaluate the relationship between hand function and objective sensory assessment found the most accurate measure was two-point discrimination (Dellon and Kallman, 1983; Novak et al., 1993a; Novak et al., 1993b). However, when examining the earliest alterations in sensibility, pressure and vibration threshold testing are the most appropriate. The results of the survey by Mielke et al. (1996) demonstrated the need to develop standardized protocols for the application of sensory tests to improve their comparability. Novak et al. (1993a) showed that static and dynamic two-point discrimination, pressure threshold with monofilaments and vibration threshold testing have a high inter-rater reliability if applied using a consistent technique.

Brief evaluations will be given of the most commonly used tests within clinical practice. Clinicians must select the most appropriate technique for individual patients.

Methods of assessment of sensation include the following:

Stereognosis
This technique assesses patients' ability to recognize common objects by touch alone. Patients must be able to manipulate an object in the hand while their vision is occluded. They should not be allowed to see the objects used for the test either before or after the assessments, thus allowing clinicians to use the same or similar objects in subsequent assessments. It may be useful to time the assessment so that on subsequent occasions the time taken to recognize a certain number of objects can be compared. The number of failures of recognition should also be noted. It is important to vary the objects used at each assessment to prevent patients from learning what to expect. At first, a selection of large objects is used, but as patients' recovery progress, the objects can be exchanged for smaller, more intricate ones.

Static and dynamic two-point discrimination
These tests require patients to identify whether they can feel one or two pressure points on their fingertips. The test can either be static, where the pressure points are applied to the skin in one place, or dynamic, where the pressure points are dragged along a digit. Dynamic two-point discrimination generally recovers before static discrimination. Patients need to identify at least seven of 10 tests correctly before discrimination at that distance can be noted as intact (Bexon and Salter, 2000).

It is important to position patients' hands in a comfortable, fully supported position so that they are able to concentrate on the test and so that the amount of pressure exerted on a digit during the examination does not create joint movement, helping patients to identify sensations. The variability of force application during the test reduces its reliability. Patients' vision is occluded and they are told to answer either *'one'* or *'two'* depending on the number of pressure points they feel. The most accurate method of applying this assessment is by the use of a discriminator (Figure 8.14). Dellon (1978) noted that during dynamic two-point discrimination testing, the prongs should be moved in a proximal to distal direction; however, this test has been criticized because of the capacity for variation in its application and lack of standardization (Ewing-Fess, 1997).

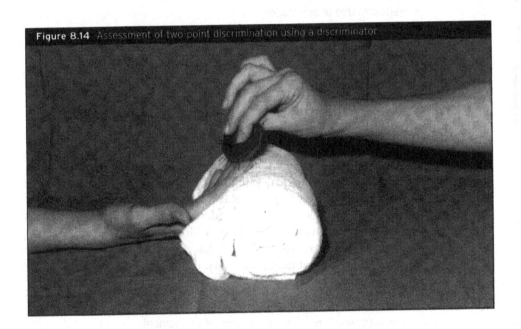

Figure 8.14 Assessment of two-point discrimination using a discriminator

Monofilaments

This method of evaluation of sensation measures deep pressure through to light touch. Graduations of filaments are applied to patients' hands. The vision is occluded and patients are asked to respond *'yes'* when they feel the stimulation. They should respond to the first stimulus if they are able to detect it; however, if they do not, the stimulus may be repeated twice more to improve the reliability of the test (Bell-Krotoski et al., 1993). It is recommended that the lightest filament be applied first, followed by the others in order until one is detected. Bell-Krotoski et al. (1993) noted that this method of application increases reliability as it minimizes patients' fatigue and distraction. The level of force that is applied is controlled by the fact that the filaments will bend when they reach their maximal force and maintain this force constantly until release (Bell-Krotoski et al., 1993). It is recommended that the filament should remain in contact with patients' skin for 1.5 seconds (Bell- Krotoski et al., 1993).

Vibration

The most commonly used method of applying a vibratory stimulus to the hand is the use of a tuning fork. However, Bell-Krotoski et al. (1993) noted their limitations in the assessment of peripheral nerves:

- application is easily varied, that is, the tip or the side of the instrument is applied
- variable force of application
- variable frequencies.

Another method of application of a vibratory force is the use of a vibrometer. Kamon (1994) described the use of a vibrometer and concluded that the vibrometer provided a reliable and valid assessment tool that can be applied in a standardized manner.

Pain

Measurement of pain is usually subjective, that is, patients describe their symptoms and apply numerical valuations of their severity. However, the way in which patients describe their pain varies between individuals. What might be termed soreness, aching or tenderness may not be considered as 'pain' to another individual. Boscheinen-Morrin and Connolly (2001) noted the importance of patients' own descriptions of their pain, which needs to include details of depth, intensity, duration, area and behaviour.

Factors affecting patients' pain include the following:

- Individual patients' personality or attitude.
- Patients' emotional state at the time of assessment.
- Individuals' motivation to mask their discomfort or overemphasize it, for example a patient who is under financial pressure to return to work attempts to conceal discomfort in order to resume greater levels of function, or patients overemphasize their symptoms in order to increase their chances of compensation after injury.
- Familial, social and cultural influences on coping with and expressing pain.
- Effective analgesia.
- Relationship with healthcare professionals.

Methods of assessment of pain include the following:

- *Pain interviews*: usually focus on the nature, location and behaviour of pain; are time-consuming.
- *Numerical rating scales*: patients are asked to describe their pain in terms of a numeric scale, either with or without a verbal description, for example percentages; these are quick and easy to use.
- *Visual analogue scale*: this is the most commonly used method of assessing pain in clinical practice. A 10-cm horizontal scale, with end-points stated as 'no pain' at the left side of the line and 'pain as bad as it can be' at the right side of the line, is presented and explained to patients. They are then required to mark a vertical line on the scale that denotes where their pain is perceived to be between these variables. The distance between the left end-point of the scale and the patient's mark can be measured to give a score. The assessment can be repeated at subsequent evaluations and compared.

The visual analogue scale has been demonstrated to be reliable (Bowsher, 1994) yet quick and easy to use (McCormack et al., 1988). Waterfield and Sim (1996) noted that its greatest strength is its potential responsiveness to change. However, in a study by Dixon and Bird (1981) it was shown that reproducibility of a set of visual analogue scales was variable, indicating the possibility of error.

Neurological

The effects of neurological injury or disease can be identified by numerous assessment methods. Loss of range of motion and muscle power has already been discussed; these could be because of injury to the motor component of the peripheral nerves of the upper limb. The specific evaluation of sensation and pain has also been described; however, further specific neurological assessments include the investigation of peripheral nerve mobility and reflexes.

Neural glide
To assess the mobility and health of the peripheral nerves in the upper limb, tension tests can be used (Butler, 1991). The application of sequential tension to the peripheral nerves by varying the positions of the peripheral joints and the spine aims to gradually produce a nerve stretch. The order in which the joints are moved is specified but can be reversed. The aims of upper limb tension tests are to identify pathology and areas of reduced neural glide. It is beyond the scope of this text to describe the application of these tests in detail but readers are referred to the work of Butler (1991).

Reflexes

The most commonly tested reflexes in the upper limb are those of biceps, triceps and brachioradialis. The reflexes should be compared on either side and Magee (1992) graded them as:

- absent
- diminished
- average
- exaggerated
- clonus.

Methods of testing neurological function include the following:

- *Biceps (C5-C6)*: the examiner places the thumb over the biceps tendon and hits the nail with the reflex hammer.
- *Triceps (C7-C8)*: the examiner hits directly over the tendon, usually with the patient's shoulder supported in abduction and internal rotation.
- *Brachioradialis (C5-C6)*: the examiner hits directly over the tendon distally.

Function

The aim of the assessment of hand function is to evaluate the activity of the upper limb as it is normally used during everyday activities. There are literally hundreds of published hand function assessments. Some assess dexterity, whereas others attempt to evaluate the integrated use of the upper limb and hand. A number of tests, such as the Jebsen hand function test (Jebsen et al., 1969), time how long it takes to complete various tasks. However, it is questionable whether the time it takes to complete a task necessarily gives any information about how well the activity is performed. More recently, patients' perception of their own function has been examined rather than relying upon physiotherapists' interpretation of findings, for example the Disabilities of the Arm, Shoulder and Hand questionnaire (DASH).

Disabilities of the Arm, Shoulder and Hand Questionnaire (DASH)

This is a patient-administered measure of symptoms and functional status with the focus on physical function. It was developed to be used by clinicians in daily practice and as a research tool (Hudak et al., 1996). The validity of the questionnaire has been demonstrated (Amadio et al., 1996; Navsarikar et al., 1999), although Beaton et al. (2001) emphasized that caution must be taken when attributing validity to an assessment tool such as the DASH as each new application of the questionnaire should be evaluated. This method of functional assessment can be used within a busy hand therapy unit because it is quick to use and reflects subjects' perceptions of their functional ability rather than physiotherapists' interpretations.

Hand functional assessments can be time-consuming. Often, we will simply ask patients what activities they are finding difficult to perform and base our treatment around their limitations. If a more detailed functional assessment is required, an appropriate test should be identified from recent literature.

Specific tests

Finklestein test
This tests for the presence of DeQuervain syndrome. The patient's thumb is passively adducted and flexed followed by a quick passive ulnar deviation of the wrist. A sharp pain experienced over the first extensor compartment containing the extensor pollicis brevis and abductor pollicis longus determines a positive response (Aulicino, 1995). A comparison with the unaffected hand should be made, as this procedure in itself can be uncomfortable.

Froment test
Patients are asked to hold a piece of paper with both hands using a lateral pinch grip, the examiner then attempts to pull the piece of paper out of the patient's grip. Normally, patients use the adductor pollicis muscle to resist the examiner, however if there is an ulnar nerve palsy the flexor pollicis longus tendon is used and the interphalangeal joint of the thumb flexes (Magee, 1992).

Phalen test
Pressure is exerted over the carpal tunnel whilst the wrist is held in flexion for at least one minute. A positive response is demonstrated if carpal tunnel symptoms are reported (Magee, 1992).

Tinel sign
Gentle tapping in a distal to proximal direction along the route of a nerve will determine how far a damaged nerve has re-grown. At the level that the nerve has reached patients will report a tingling or electric shock sensation elicited by the tapping (Magee, 1992). As a regenerating nerve progresses distally the tip is hypersensitive, therefore any stimulus produces neural signs, such as 'pins and needles' (Irwin, 1999). The Tinel test can also be used over areas in which nerves may be being compressed, for example at the carpal tunnel.

Tactile adherence test

A plastic pen is dragged along the surface of patients' skin. If sweating is present, a resistance to movement will be felt. If there is no resistance, there could be a loss of the nerve supply therefore reducing the action of the sweat glands (Harrison, 1974).

Intrinsic tightness test

The metacarpophalangeal joint is held in extension and passive flexion of the proximal interphalangeal joint is attempted. A positive result is demonstrated if there is resistance to the proximal interphalangeal joint flexion with the metacarpophalangeal joint in extension caused by shortening of the intrinsic muscles (van Veldhoven, 2000).

Psychological

In the initial weeks after injury, it is not unusual for patients to report symptoms of post-traumatic stress disorder. However, if these persist they can seriously affect recovery both physically and psychologically. Indicative signs of psychological distress, such as flashbacks of the accident, anxiety and grief have been demonstrated as early as on admission to the Accident and Emergency Department (Grunert et al., 1992). Although it is not within the realm of physiotherapists to provide counselling, in order for physiotherapy staff to make an appropriate referral to other professionals it is necessary that they are able to recognize the signs of psychological distress.

Nichols (1984) developed a four-part model of care that is a useful framework for physiotherapists to work within. The first part is emotional care: physiotherapists should demonstrate empathy and understanding by listening and encouraging patients to verbalize their feelings. Next is informational care: physiotherapistshould give clear, accurate information in a manner that is acceptable to individual patients. Excellent communication skills are necessary to achieve this, and the information given may need to be repeated on subsequent occasions until full understanding and acceptance is achieved. The third part of the Nichol (1984) model is basic counselling, and the most important stage, monitoring or referral on to professional psychological help, follows this.

The future

Methods of hand assessment are changing and progressing constantly. It is the duty of physiotherapists to keep abreast of the changes and critically evaluate new methods to ensure that they are reliable and valid. In this era of advancements in technology, the use of computer technology will be embraced by physiotherapists, and may provide opportunities to make accurate assessments that are quick to measure. However, as with any assessments these methods must be monitored strictly to ensure their accuracy. Murray and Simpson (1998) and Simpson et al. (1999) demonstrated this in their reports of the development of the Hand Assessment and Treatment System (HATS).

Documentation

Accurate, legible documentation of the results obtained from assessment is fundamental to comparison of subsequent assessments and appropriate treatment planning and goal-setting. Lengthy descriptions of findings should be replaced with clear diagrams and complicated lists of data can be tabulated. A number of 'ready to use' assessment sheets are available. Despite the advantage of standardizing the order of assessment, in clinical practice these assessment forms can be limiting as they can inhibit the natural progression of evaluation. They are most useful to inexperienced staff who require a guide and prompt to their examinations. However, as staff gain experience and confidence they may lose their relevance in clinical practice.

Outcome measures

It has been established that assessment is an essential part of hand physiotherapy. A progression of this would be the widespread use of standardized outcome measures to enable physiotherapists to compare treatment methods more accurately. At the Fourth Congress of the International Federation of Societies for Hand Therapy in 1998, a workshop was organized to examine the issue of outcome codes (Glover, 1998). At this workshop outcome measures were categorized into:

- patient-orientated outcomes
- disease, disorder or region-specific instruments
- physical performance measures
- functional tests of performance.

Macey and Burke (1995) noted that outcome measures should be objective, although some subjective factors will influence outcome:

- psychological aspects
- individual motivation
- cosmesis
- compensation claims
- patient satisfaction.

Further reading

Macey AC, Burke FDJ (1995) Outcome of hand surgery. Journal of Hand Surgery 20B(6): 841-5.

References

Allen EVJ (1929) Thromboangitis obliterans: methods of diagnosis of chronic occlusive arterial lesions distal to the wrist with illustrative cases. American Journal of Medical Science 78: 237.

Amadio P, Beaton D, Bombadier C, Davis A, Hawker G, Hudak P et al. (1996) Measuring disability and symptoms of the upper limb: a validation study of the DASH questionnaire. Orlando, FL: American College of Rheumatology 60th National Scientific Meeting.

American Society for Surgery of the Hand (ASSH) (1976) The Hand - Examination and Diagnosis. Colorado: Aurora.

Ashbell TS, Kutz JE, Kleinert HE (1967) The digital Allen test. Plastic and Reconstructive Surgery 39(3): 311-12.

Aulicino PLI (1995) Clinical examination of the hand. In: JM Hunter, EJ Mackin, AD Callahan (eds) Rehabilitation of the Hand, Vol 1. St Louis, MI: Mosby.

Baryza MJ, Baryza GA (1995) The Vancouver scar scale: an administration tool and its interrater reliability. Journal of Burn Care and Rehabilitation 6(5): 535-8.

Beaton DE, Davis AM, Hudak P, McConnell S (2001) The DASH (Disabilities of the Arm, Shoulder and Hand) outcome measure: what do we know about it now? British Journal of Hand Therapy 6(4): 109-18.

Bechtol C (1954) Grip test: the use of a dynamometer with adjustable hand spacings. Journal of Bone and Joint Surgery 38A: 82-4.

Bell-Krotoski JA, Weinstein S, Weinstein C (1993) Testing sensibility, including touch - pressure, two-point discrimination, point localisation and vibration. Journal of Hand Therapy Apr-Jun: 114-23.

Bell-Krotoski JA, Berger Lee DE, Beach RB (1995) Hand volume measurement. In: JM Hunter, EJ Mackin, AD Callahan (eds) Rehabilitation of the Hand, Vol 1. St Louis, MI: Mosby.

Bexon C, Salter M (2000) Assessment. In: JM Hunter, EJ Mackin, AD Callahan (eds) Rehabilitation of the Hand, Vol 1. St Louis, MI: Mosby.

Boland R, Adams R (1996) Development and evaluation of a precision forearm and hand volumeter and measuring cylinder. Journal of Hand Therapy 9(4): 349-58.

Boone DC, Azen SP, Lin CM (1978) Reliability of goniometric measurements. Physical Therapy 58: 1355-60.

Boscheinen-Morrin J, Davey V, Connolly WB (1992) The Hand: Fundamentals of Therapy (second edition). Oxford: Butterworth-Heinemann.

Boscheinen-Morrin J, Connolly WB (2001) The Hand: Fundamentals of Therapy (third edition). Oxford: Butterworth-Heinemann.

Bowling A (1997) Research Methods in Health, Investigating Health and Health Services. Buckingham: Open University Press.

Bowsher D (1994) Acute and chronic pain and assessment. In: PE Wells, V Frampton, D Bowsher (eds) Pain Management by Physiotherapy (second edition). Oxford: Butterworth-Heinemann.

Boyes JH (1950) Flexor tendon grafts in the finger and thumb, an evaluation of end results. Journal of Bone and Joint Surgery 32A: 489-99.

Bruton A, Ellis B, Goddard J (1999) Comparison of visual estimation and goniometry for assessment of metacarpophalangeal joint angle. Physiotherapy 85(4): 201-8.

Butler D (1991) Mobilisation of the Nervous System. London: Churchill Livingstone.

Callahan AD (1995) Sensibility assessment: prerequisites and techniques for nerve lesions in continuity and nerve lacerations In: In: JM Hunter, EJ Mackin, AD Callahan (eds) Rehabilitation of the Hand, Vol 1. St Louis, MI: Mosby.

Cederlund R (1998) Hand assessment in a Swedish hand rehabilitation unit. British Journal of Hand Therapy) 3(2):9-10.

Collings J (1997) A handy tip - Kapandji's thumb opposition evaluation. British Journal of Hand Therapy 2(6): 16.

Cyriax J (1982) Textbook of Orthopaedic Medicine, Vol 1, Diagnosis of Soft Tissue Lesions (eighth edition). London: Baillière Tindall.

Dellon AL (1978) The moving two-point discrimination test: clinical evaluation of the quickly adapting fibre/receptor system. Journal of Hand Surgery (Am) 3: 474-81.

Dellon AL, Kallman W (1983) Evaluation of functional sensation in the hand. Journal of Hand Surgery (Am) 8: 865-70.

Dixon JS, Bird A (1981) Reproducibility along a 10 cm vertical visual analogue scale. Annals of Rheumatic Diseases 40: 87-9.

Ellis B, Bruton AJ (1998) Clinical assessment of the hand - a review of joint angle measures. British Journal of Hand Therapy 3(2): 5-8.

Ewing-Fess E (1995) Documentation: essential element of an upper extremity assessment battery. In: JM Hunter, EJ Mackin, AD Callahan (eds) Rehabilitation of the Hand, Vol 1. St Louis, MI: Mosby.

Ewing-Fess E (1997) Human performance: an appropriate measure of instrument reliability. Journal of Hand Therapy 10: 46-7.

Firrell JC, Crain GM (1996) Which setting of the dynamometer provides maximal grip strength? Journal of Hand Surgery, 21A: 397-401.

Gilbertson L, Barber-Lomax S (1994) Power and pinch grip strength recorded using the hand held Jamar dynamometer and B+L pinch gauge: British normative data for adults. British Journal of Occupational Therapy 57(12): 483-8.

Glover M (1998) Reports from the Fourth Congress of the International Federation of Societies for Hand Therapy, Vancouver, Canada, 1998: outcome measures. British Journal of Hand Therapy 3(4): 24-5.

Goldsmith N, Juzi E (1998) Inter-rater reliability of two trainer rater using a goniometer for the measurement of finger joints. British Journal of Hand Therapy 3(2):11-12.

Grigsgy de Linde L, Miles WK (1995) Remodeling of scar tissue in the burned hand. In: JM Hunter, EJ Mackin, AD Callahan (eds) Rehabilitation of the Hand, Vol 1. St Louis, MI: Mosby.

Grunert BK, Devine CA, Smith CJ, Matloub HS, Sanger JR, Yousif NJ (1992) Graded work exposure to promote work return after severe hand trauma: a replicated study? Annals of Plastic Surgery 29(6): 532-6.

Harrison SH (1974) The tactile adherence test estimating loss of sensation after nerve injury. The Hand 6(2): 148-9.

Hellibrandt FA, Duvall EN, Moore MLJ (1949) The measurement of joint motion part III – reliability of goniometry. Physical Therapy Review 29: 32-7.

Hildreth DH, Breidenbach WC (1989) Detection of submaximal effort by the use of rapid exchange grip. Journal of Hand Surgery 14A: 747-50.

Hudak PL, Amadio PC, Bombardier C (1996) Development of an upper extremity outcome measure: the DASH (disabilities of the arm, shoulder and hand). American Journal of Industrial Medicine 29: 602-8.

Irwin MS (1999) Nerve repair and regeneration. British Journal of Hand Therapy 4(1): 8-12.

Jebsen RH, Taylor N, Trieschmann RB, Trotter MJ, Howard LA (1969) An objective and standardized test of hand function. Archives of Physical Medicine and Rehabilitation June: 311-20.

Kaltenborn FM (1980) Mobilisation of the Extremity Joints. Oslo: Olaf Norlis.

Kamon N (1994) Quantitative measurement of vibratory perception threshold using a new vibrometer TM-31A. Journal of Occupational Medicine 36(9): 989-96.

Kapandji A (1992) Clinical evaluation of the thumb's opposition. Journal of Hand Therapy Apr-Jun: 102-6.

King T (1993) The effect of water temperature on hand volume during volumetric measurement using the water displacement method. Journal of Hand Therapy 6(3): 202-4.

Lamb DW (1987) The Paralysed Hand. London: Churchill Livingstone.

Macey AC, Burke F (1995) Outcome of hand surgery. Journal of Hand Surgery 20B(6): 841-55.

Magee DJ (1992) Orthopaedic Physical Assessment (second edition). London: WB Saunders.

Maithiowetz V (1991) Reliability and validity of grip and pinch strength. Critical review. Rehabilitative Medicine 2: 201-13.

Maitland G (1992) Peripheral Manipulation (eighth edition). Edinburgh: Churchill Livingstone.

McCormack HM, Home DJ de L, Sheather S (1988) Clinical applications of visual analogue scales: a critical review. Psychological Medicine 18: 1007-19.

Mielke K, Novak CB, Mackinnon SE, Feely CA (1996) Hand sensibility measures used by therapists. Annals of Plastic Surgery 36(3): 292-6.

Moore ML. (1949) The measurement of joint motion part II - the technique of goniometry. Physical Therapy Review 29: 256-64.

Murray K, Simpson C (1998) A therapist view of the hats project? British Journal of Hand Therapy 3(2): 13.

Navsarikar A, Gladman DD, Husted JA, Cook RJ (1999) Validity assessment of the disabilities of arm, shoulder and hand questionnaire (DASH) for patients with psoriatic arthritis. Journal of Rheumatology 26 (10): 2191-4.

Ng GYF, Fan ACC (2001) Does elbow position affect strength and reproducibility of power grip measurements? Physiotherapy 87(2): 68-72.

Nicholas JS (1977) The swollen hand. Physiotherapy 63(9): 285-6.

Nichols K (1984) Psychological Care in Physical Illness. London: Croom Helm.

Novak CB, Mackinson SE, Williams JI, Kelly L (1993a) Establishment of reliability in the evaluation of hand sensibility? Plastic Reconstructive Surgery 92: 311-22.

Novak CB, Kelly L, Mackinson SE (1993b) Correlation of two-point discrimination and hand function following median nerve injury. Annals of Plastic Surgery 31: 495-8.

Pratt AL, Burr NJ (2001) A review of goniometry use within current hand therapy practice. British Journal of Hand Therapy 6(2): 45-9.

Richards LG, Olson B, Palmiter-Thomas P (1996) How forearm position affects grip strength. American Journal of Occupational Therapy 50: 133-8.

Salter M (1987) Hand Injuries: A Therapeutic Approach. London: Churchill Livingstone.

Sawada Y (1994) A method of recording and objective assessment of hypertrophic burn scars. Burns 20(1): 76-8.

Simpson C, Murray K, Topping M, Perlick O, Bolmsjo G, Wicksramasinghe Y et al. (1999) The development of a clinical evaluation protocol for use with a computerised hand assessment system: preliminary findings. British Journal of Hand Therapy 4(2): 68-73.

Solgaard S, Carlsen A, Kramhoft M (1986) Reproducibility of goniometry of the wrist. Scandinavian Journal of Rehabilitative Medicine 18: 5-7.

Sorenson MK (1989) The edematous hand. Physical Therapy 69(12): 1059-64.

Stokes HM, Landrieu KW, Domangue B, Kunen S (1995) Identification of low-effort patients through dynamometry. Journal of Hand Surgeryi 20A: 1047-56.

van Veldhoven G (2000) Intrinsic and extrinsic tightness - the importance of the pre- splint test to determine MCP inclusion and position in orthotics. British Journal of Hand Therapy 5(3): 75-6.

Vasiliauskas R, Dijkers M, Buda Abela M, Lundgren L (1995) Characteristics in addition to size of the contralateral hand predict hand volume but are not clinically useful. Journal of Hand Therapy 8(4): 258-63.

Wagner C (1977) Determination of the rotatory flexibility of the elbow joint. European Journal of Applied Physiology 37: 47-50.

Waterfield J, Sim J (1996) Clinical assessment of pain by the visual analogue sealer. British Journal of Therapy and Rehabilitation 3(2): 94-7.

Chapter 9

Treatment modalities

Introduction

> The hand therapist plays a critical role in preventing, monitoring and treating complications. (Azad et al., 2001)

Although most of this chapter is related to hand therapy, the principles of treatment can be related to any plastic surgery procedure whether it be after a burn injury or an elective breast reconstruction. It is not the intention of this book to give prescriptive regimes for individual injuries or surgery. Physiotherapists are only too aware that, in clinical practice, patients never fit these categories. Therefore, by accurate assessment and identification of problems and priorities it is anticipated that physiotherapists will be able to select appropriate treatment modalities to address their findings, based on their anatomical and pathological knowledge. Essentially, patients should be treated as individuals (Barillo et al., 1997).

Physiotherapists cannot work in isolation, they need to gain patients' trust and compliance through education, reassurance, support and encouragement; they need the support of the medical team and other specialist professionals, and communication is a vital component of this teamwork (Jefferis and Dickinson, 1998). Each profession should complement another and overlap slightly to achieve the ultimate goal – optimal patient recovery.

The following treatment modalities should be selected for their suitability at each stage of patients' recovery. The aim of all of them is to complement and assist the body's natural healing processes while preventing complications. It is essential for physiotherapists to understand and recognize the stages of tissue healing (*see* Chapter 1) in order to promote healing and identify complications or improvements.

Education

Patient education is fundamental to therapeutic intervention. If patients understand their injury, surgery or condition, and understand why they are asked to follow a specific treatment programme, be it a particular exercise or to wear a particular splint, they are more likely to comply (Groth and Wulf, 1995). Clear, concise explanations of pathology and treatment, in a way that does not patronize patients, are required. Providing written instructions illustrated with diagrams may also assist patient recall.

However, it is not only patients who need educating about treatment; everyone involved with them needs to be educated as well – carers, therapists, doctors, nurses and employers (Ashe, 2001). Everyone involved in supporting patients should encourage them and facilitate their rehabilitation towards agreed goals. Patients are at the centre of the team approach to care and it is imperative that they are encouraged to take an active part in their own rehabilitation (Ashe, 2001) and the decisions that affect them.

In addition to educating patients about their condition or injury and explaining why treatments that are recommended are necessary, it is the responsibility of physiotherapists to assist patients in complying with their treatment programmes. For example, splints should be made as comfortable as possible, and strategies to remind patients to exercise or use an affected digit should be suggested.

Parsley (1998) emphasized the need for education, support and encouragement, but warned that dependency should be avoided. Education should facilitate independence, and patients should be encouraged to accept responsibility for their own treatment and recovery. Factors that influence compliance include:

- patient-therapist relationship
- level of patient understanding
- cultural
- financial
- level of patient motivation
- patient recall
- perceived benefits.

Further reading

Groth GN, Wulf MB (1995) Compliance with hand rehabilitation: health beliefs and strategies. Journal of Hand Therapy 8(1): 18-22.

Wound care

Many patients treated by physiotherapists have open wounds. Although responsibility for the management of these wounds is usually directed by nursing staff, it is part of the role of physiotherapists to monitor wounds for signs of improvement or deterioration, and to prevent infection by the use of aseptic techniques.

Traditionally, sterile saline has been used to irrigate and cleanse wounds. However, in a study by Angeras et al. (1992) it was found that the use of tap water had no detrimental effects on healing when compared with the use of saline and this method of cleansing wounds has now been accepted in general practice (Oliver, 1997).

Elevation

The most commonly used and effective method of managing oedema is elevation of the hand (Landsmeer, 1974; Williams, 1980). All patients with hand injuries or those who have had hand surgery should elevate their hands. The only exception to this rule concerns injuries in which the vascular supply to the hand is compromised, for example replantations.

Elevation utilizes the effects of gravity. Gravity increases the rate of venous and lymphatic drainage, reduces hydrostatic pressure in the vessels and therefore reduces the rate of oedema formation (Parsley, 1998; Palmada et al., 1999). Ideally, the hand should be raised above shoulder height (Sorenson, 1989; Palmada et al., 1999). However, careful observation is necessary to ensure there is no evidence of vascular insufficiency or nerve compression. Sorenson (1989) suggested that the use of slings should be avoided as they can cause a blockage to drainage. Sorenson (1989) also noted that patients should maintain the hand above the level of the right atrium when sitting and put the hand on the head when walking – although compliance with this posture was not investigated.

Elevation should be combined with the whole treatment package to achieve optimal reduction of oedema. The resolution of oedema can be enhanced further by the addition of active exercise while positioned in elevation (Collings, 1999) to utilize the effects of the muscle pump.

Active exercise

Palmada et al. (1999) summarized the effects of active exercise as increasing blood flow and producing a muscle pump, thereby reducing oedema, maintaining soft tissue extensibility (in particular tendon glide) and increasing the healing plus the strength of damaged tissues. However, there needs to be a balance between exercise to achieve the benefits listed below, and rest to allow resolution of inflammation and prevention of increased pain and swelling (*see* Chapter 7). The aims of active exercise are to:

- *Reduce oedema*: active exercise is the most effective way of reducing oedema (Sorenson, 1989). Both venous and lymphatic drainage are increased with active exercise; however, Sorenson (1989) did warn against simply 'wiggling' the fingers as a strong contraction with full range motion is necessary to force fluid out of hand. Simons et al. (1996) advocated the use of isometric abduction and adduction exercises in the hand to produce a deep muscle pump, thereby reducing oedema. To obtain the best results active exercises are performed in elevation.

- *Maintain or restore joint range of motion*: isolated joint active exercises are most effective in maintaining or restoring range of motion in the acutely injured hand. However, once the initial inflammatory period has passed combined active exercises are necessary to achieve the full diversity of motion of the hand.

- *Maintain or restore soft tissue extensibility*: the beneficial effects of active exercise after flexor tendon repairs have been established (Gelberman et al., 1983; Cullen et al., 1989; Small et al., 1989). In this situation the use of active exercise early in the rehabilitative process aims to prevent adhesions, maintain tendon glide and increase the tensile strength of the repairs. Silverskjold et al. (1992) demonstrated that active motion after flexor tendon repair was 90% more effective at achieving tendon gliding than passive joint motion at the proximal interphalangeal joint. Early active regimes for extensor tendons are also being developed for the same reasons as they were developed for flexors, that is, to prevent adhesions or increase tensile strength, etc. (Ip and Chow, 1997; Ranelli, 1998; Hunt, 2000).

- *Prevent or adapt interstructural adhesions*: if oedema is present within the hand after an injury or surgery there is a risk that structures lying in close proximity may become adhered to each other. These interstructural adhesions will prevent normal gliding and therefore reduce range of motion. To prevent this, active exercise is incorporated into treatment regimes but to ensure that all of the structures are moved against their neighbours (differential glide) rather than moving with them, the four main types of grip patterns should be used (Figure 9.1): hook; full; straight; flat. Isolated joint exercises (blocking exercises) also produce differential glide of tendons within the hand, for example differential glide of the flexor digitorum profundus tendon is achieved by immobilizing the metacarpophalangeal and proximal interphalangeal joints of a digit whilst actively flexing the distal interphalangeal joint (Figure 9.2). Active mobilization aids maintenance of neural gliding and excursion after a nerve repair in the same way as it does after tendon repairs. Normally, nerve excursion is 3.5 cm for the median nerve and 1 cm for digital nerves; however, if a nerve becomes tethered it can cause hypersensitivity (Irwin, 1999).

Figure 9.1 Grip postures: (a) hook; (b) full; (c) straight; (d) flat

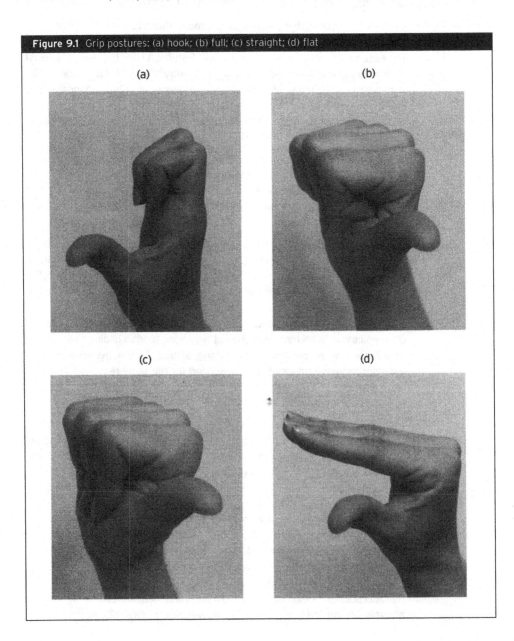

(a)

(b)

(c)

(d)

Figure 9.2 Blocking exercises

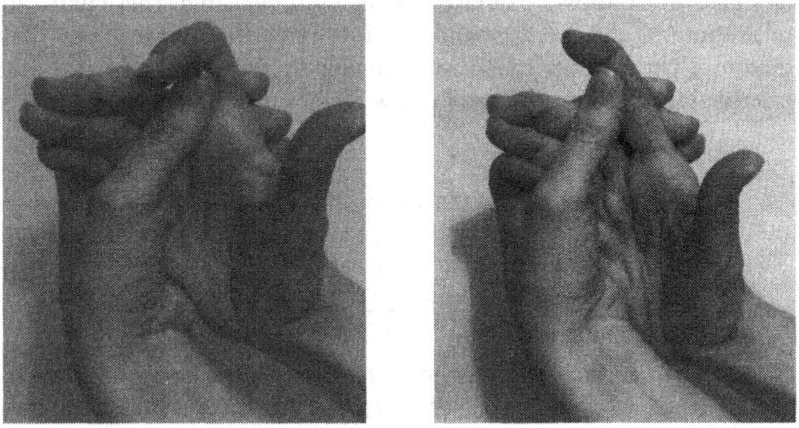

- *Maintain or restore muscle power*: although isometric exercise will increase muscle power, concentric and eccentric muscle contraction is necessary to achieve optimal strength.
- *Maintain normal patterns of motion*: patients rarely appreciate the patterns of motion within the hand. In fact, it is not uncommon for patients to 'forget' how they previously moved their hand to achieve full range of motion or a particular function. Patients may need to re-learn movement patterns and these should be re-established as soon as possible to prevent adaptation (Collings, 1999).
- *Aid tissue healing*: connective tissue healing is promoted with application of moderate levels of stress (Hildebrand and Frank, 1998). Early application of motion also encourages the development of scar tissue in linear patterns that follow the lines of stress (Salter and Bexon, 2000).
- *Restore function*: the resumption of joint range of motion through active exercise facilitates the restoration of functional activities. However, an absolute full range of active joint motion is not necessary for patients to be fully functional.

A sound knowledge of normal hand anatomy will assist the selection and grading of active exercise. For example, after a mallet injury (division of the extensor tendon at its insertion to the base of the distal phalanx) the distal interphalangeal joint is immobilized for approximately six weeks. On removal of the immobilizing splint, active distal interphalangeal joint flexion is understandably limited but starting distal interphalangeal joint blocking exercises (*see* Figure 9.2 above) may apply too much strain to the still-delicate repair site. Therefore, active hook fist (*see* Figure 9.1 above) exercises can be used instead as these will allow the relaxation of the lateral bands of the extensor digitorum tendon (and therefore the tendon repair site) owing to the flexion of the proximal interphalangeal joint, but still allow distal interphalangeal joint flexion.

Precautions:

- The rate and timing of the introduction of active exercise depends on the particular structures that have been injured, on confidence in any repairs and on the reaction of individual patients.
- Aggressive active exercises are contraindicated if infection is present (Salter and Bexon, 2000).
- After reconstructive surgery with grafts or flaps, active exercise should be practised under the guidance of physiotherapists so that grafts and anastomoses can be protected from damage (Ranelli et al., 2000).
- Physiotherapists may need to compromise the amount of joint range of motion that they attempt to achieve. For example there is little benefit in achieving full extension in the joints of the digits at the cost of flexion as for a hand to be used functionally, joint flexion is paramount.
- When treating hands after injuries or surgery, active exercises must be given for all the joints of the upper limb rather than just the hand, as the elbow and in particular the shoulder, are also at risk of loss of motion.

Each hand therapy unit will have a variety of active exercise treatment protocols for specific injuries, for example flexor tendon and extensor tendon regimes. The regimes are usually adapted from those reported in the literature and are developed with reference to the particular client base, or surgeons' or physiotherapists' preferences.

Passive movements

Maitland (1991) described passive physiological movements as rhythmical movements at varying levels of range of motion (*mobilizations*), or as overpressure or *stretch* at end of range of motion.

Passive movements or mobilizations

Large-amplitude mobilizations are used in pain-free ranges of normal joint physiological motion to utilize pain gate mechanisms (Melzack and

Wall, 1965; Chester and Davies, 2001). After this, if there is no alteration in range of motion, the mobilizations may need to be increased into the painful range, or accessory mobilizations may be incorporated into the treatment (Chester and Davies, 2001).

The aims of passive movements or mobilizations are to:

- maintain joint range of motion
- increase joint range of motion (Chester and Davies, 2001)
- prevent joint and soft tissue contractures (Ranelli et al., 2000)
- maintain muscle extensibility (Ranelli et al., 2000).

Overly aggressive passive mobilizations performed during the inflammatory phase of tissue healing will exacerbate pain and oedema. However, the incorporation of passive mobilizations early in the fibroplastic phase of tissue healing (*see* Chapter 1) will facilitate the maintenance of scar length, as at this stage the collagen is still malleable (Azad et al., 2000).

Passive mobilizations are particularly useful before active exercises as they reduce joint stiffness and therefore facilitate a greater range of active motion (Boscheinen-Morrin and Conolly, 2001). They are vital after a peripheral nerve injury to maintain joint motion that can no longer be achieved actively.

Passive stretch

A passive stretch is applied to scar tissue to attempt to elongate the scar. The stretch should be applied slowly and gently (Herndon, 1996) while the physiotherapist observes the scar tissue for blanching, as this indicates that the stretch is being effective. The stretch should be held at the end of the available range for a few seconds but should not be overly uncomfortable for the patient. A combined passive stretch of all the joints of the limb will create an effective stretch to all the soft tissues. Passive stretching can be administered by physiotherapists, patients themselves, or via splintage (*see below*). An excellent method of applying a passive stretch to the digits to produce joint flexion is to use strapping, a flexion glove or a boxing glove bandage.

Precautions:

- Passive motion will not aid the dispersal of oedema, in fact, it may increase the extent of swelling if it is painful and increases inflammation (Sorenson, 1989).
- Passive movements may need to be avoided in patients who are suffering with complex regional pain syndrome as they can exacerbate the symptoms (Parsley, 1998).

Accessory movements

Accessory movements are small intra-articular gliding movements that occur during normal joint motion but cannot be reproduced actively, for example rotation at the metacarpophalangeal joints of the fingers during strong gripping of a spherical object.

The directions of motion are:

- rotation
- distraction
- compression
- lateral glide
- medial glide
- anteroposterior glide (AP)
- posteroanterior glide (PA)
- abduction
- adduction.

In clinical practice, accessory mobilizations are used to assess joint integrity and to increase joint range of motion, increase circulation, aid healing and reduce pain. The directions of accessory mobilizations that are chosen for treatment are those that best relieve or reproduce patients' symptoms (Maitland, 1991).

Neural mobilization

Like any soft tissue, nerves are mobile and will glide between their adjacent structures during joint motion. Therefore, nerves are also at risk of becoming tethered by adhesions after trauma. Neural tissue is notorious for its irritability, and overmanipulation will result in an increase of neural signs, for example burning or shooting pains, or parasthesia.

Treatment modalities that aim to mobilize neural tissue:

- mobilize the surrounding tissues, for example mobilize joints with passive or accessory movements; mobilize soft tissues with massage
- mobilize the neural tissue at a site away from where the patient experiences the symptoms for example active shoulder exercises with distal joints in varying positions to achieve gentle neural stretch
- mobilize neural tissue at the site of symptoms.

Continuous passive motion

The use of continuous passive motion machines is well documented to facilitate the restoration of joint motion in the lower limb. However, continuous passive motion can also be utilized in hand therapy for injuries ranging from ligamentous injuries of the wrist (Otthiers, 1998) to hand burns (Barillo et al., 1997).

The aims of continuous passive motion are to:

- aid healing
- aid regeneration of articular structures
- prevent loss of joint range of motion
- restore joint range of motion
- reduce pain

(Salter, 1996).

However, continuous passive motion machines are costly, difficult to use for inexperienced physiotherapists, difficult to clean between patients and only provide gross ranges of motion rather than normal patterns of movement. Covey et al. (1988) performed a small study on the use of continuous passive motion with hand burns but found no difference in pain, range of motion or skin graft loss between the groups that received treatment with a continuous passive motion machine and those that did not.

Massage

The use of massage by physiotherapists has been out of vogue in recent years; however, physiotherapists are beginning to use this treatment modality again and are finding its effects surprisingly beneficial. Galley and Forster (1987) listed the beneficial effects of massage:

- soothing
- mobilizes soft tissues
- mobilizes scar tissue
- breaks down adhesions
- desensitizes
- improves skin condition and cosmesis.

Scar massage

Within burns and plastic surgery, the use of massage to modify scar tissue has long been established. However, there is little evidence to support the beneficial effects claimed as a result of the practice. Scar massage after burn injuries aims to:

- prevent adherence of the skin to the underlying structures
- reduce redness
- reduce elevation of scar
- relieve itching (pruritis)
- moisturize.

However, in a study by Patino et al. (1999), into the use of massage for hypertrophic scarring, no difference in vascularity, pliability or height of the scar was found despite its common use. Patino et al. (1999) did note, however, that pruritis was reported to decrease with massage. Other authors have investigated the use of creams when massaging scars. The aims of using cream while massaging are to reduce friction and to moisturize scars that no longer have a normal lubricating function, for example after split skin grafting (Azad et al., 2000; Gollup, 2002). Jenkins (1986) studied the use of vitamin E cream compared with aqueous cream during massage, but found no difference in scar size or range of joint motion. However, patients often report a relief of itching after massage with cream (Gollup, 2002), and they are recommended to massage three times a day after split skin grafting.

Field et al. (1998) demonstrated that the use of massage in burn-injured patients decreased anxiety, depression, anger and pain, although exactly how this worked was not understood. Otthiers (1998) also noted that massage was effective for relief of pain, aided the resolution of skin problems, was relaxing for patients and therefore facilitated rapport and promoted a better approach to rehabilitation.

Ronon (2001) examined massage in hand therapy at each stage of tissue healing as follows.

- *Inflammation:* overzealous massage could potentially cause disturbance to fibril formation, increasing fibrin production and therefore increasing scar tissue. However, it can be hypothesized that gentle massage around the injured area will decrease oedema and increase blood supply, although there is no published evidence of this.

- *Fibroplasia:* to aid collagen alignment, the healing tissue should be placed under some amount of stress or tension (*see* Chapter 1). This stress or tension can be applied by massage. Initially, gentle massage can be used as inflammation and proliferation overlap. Gradually, as tissue healing progresses, massage can be increasingly aggressive. Massage in the form of transverse frictions is particularly useful to decrease interstitial adhesions; however, stress along the line of normal motion is also necessary to align collagen. In addition to scar massage, retrograde massage can be used during fibroplasia to decrease oedema.

- *Remodelling*: massage should be aggressive and include prolonged stretching in order to minimize adhesions and contraction. Rupture of adhesions should be avoided as this would result in a recurrence of inflammation. The aim of massage should be to cause gradual minute breakdown of scar tissue.

Precautions

Overzealous scar massage on newly formed skin can be detrimental and cause wound breakdown. If used too early in the tissue-healing process, massage can increase scar tissue formation by stimulating fibroblasts (Azad et al., 2000).

Retrograde massage

The aim of retrograde massage is to reduce oedema. If used in elevation and performed from distal to proximal, retrograde massage can aid venous return, increase lymphatic drainage and mobilize fluid (Sorenson, 1989; Parsley, 1998; Palmada et al., 1999). However, it is important that after retrograde massage the dispersal of oedema is maintained by patient compliance with elevation, pressure garments and exercise. Palmada et al. (1999) also suggested that massage aids the rapport between patients and physiotherapists because of the personal contact, and helps to facilitate patients' acceptance of their injury or condition.

Compression

Compression is most commonly used to resolve oedema, but it can also be used via pressure garments to conform scars and maintain joint range of motion.

Compression for oedema

Simons et al. (1996) demonstrated that when compression was applied to the hand it activated the venous systems, therefore aiding venous drainage and oedema resolution. Sorenson (1989) noted that the application of compression after therapeutic intervention maintained the reduction in oedema that had been achieved. Palmada et al. (1999) explained the mechanism of how compression reduces oedema: the pressure within the blood vessels is increased; this in turn increases capillary filling, which facilitates reabsorption of excess interstitial fluid.

Compression should be applied in a distal to proximal direction to push the excess fluid into the lymphatic and venous systems (Palmada et al., 1999). Methods of applying compression in order to control oedema include:

- dressings
- 'off the shelf' compression dressings, gloves or sleeves, for example Coban or Tubigrip
- tailormade pressure garments
- pneumatic devices – these work in the same way as the body's muscle pump and are most effective in acute oedema (Palmada et al., 1999); they are generally ineffective for fibrosing oedema (Sorenson, 1989)
- string wrapping, either string or a narrow strip of Coban is spiralled down the digit (distal to proximal) to push oedema out of the digit and aid reabsorption.

The use of tailormade pressure garments for oedema may be costly. Their efficiency in reducing oedema means that they will need to be changed for smaller sizes regularly. A more cost-effective method is to use the 'off the shelf' gloves.

Compression for scar management

Despite the lack of evidence of their effectiveness, or knowledge of their exact mechanism of action (Staley and Richard, 1997), pressure garments are used almost routinely to modify scars after burn injuries. Pressure garments can also be used on any hypertrophic scarring or over bulky flaps (Ranelli et al., 2000).

Azad et al. (2000) presented three theories of how pressure garments modify scars:

- they occlude the vasculature in the scar, leading to hypoxia and a resultant degeneration of fibroblasts, so preventing excessive scarring
- they raise the temperature of skin, which increases collagenase activity (Quinn, 1987)
- the decreased blood supply reduces macroglobulin levels and increases collagenase activity.

Healed wounds often look acceptable initially but 3–4 weeks later they may begin to become hypertrophic as the collagen becomes more extensive and forms whorls followed by scar contraction (Appleby, 1997). The aims of pressure garments are to:

- maintain the flat appearance of a scar (Appleby, 1997)
- relieve itching that is common during scar maturation
- protect fragile skin from minor trauma and sunlight
- allow continuation of exercise and activities of daily living.

Pressure garments can be fitted immediately after a wound has healed, in an attempt to prevent the development of hypertrophic scarring, or as soon as signs of hypertrophy are seen, which is usually within 3 months of healing (Appleby, 1997). Hayakawa et al. (1977) suggested that pressure garments should be fitted as early as 2 weeks after grafting. To be effective pressure garments must be custom-made and worn for 23 hours a day for at least 6 months (Azad et al., 2000), but ideally for up to 2 years after injury. Gollup (2002) recommended the application of a continuous pressure of 25 mmHg via the pressure garment. To encourage compliance with the use of pressure garments patients and their carers need to be educated about why they are needed (Ranelli et al., 2000). The use of different-coloured garments may increase compliance (Thompson et al., 1992) especially in children. However, pressure garments can only control scarring, they do not cure it (Ward, 1991) and, if not carefully monitored, they can also produce some undesired effects:

- skin breakdown
- web space discomfort
- inconvenience
- difficulty with personal hygiene

(Clarke et al., 1997).

Pressure garments applied to the hand should leave the fingertips free to facilitate function and sensation. Although the garments give a slight resistance to motion, they should not restrict joint movement. Inserts are sometimes used beneath the pressure garments to fill anatomical concavities where it is difficult to apply pressure.

Despite their frequent use, and numerous reports of their benefits from patients and in the literature, Chang et al. (1995) found no significant difference in scar maturation using the Vancouver Burn Scar Assessment Scale as an assessment tool (see Chapter 8) when comparing the use of pressure therapy with no pressure. In addition, Mann et al. (1997) studied pressure garment–scar interface pressures and found inconsistent pressures.

Compression to maintain joint range of motion

Soft tissue deformities that are passively correctable but are maintained out of habit can be corrected by increasing the pressure to the opposing aspect of a joint, for example applying a garment that has a reinforced lycra band on the extensor aspect to prevent flexion deformity (Clarke et al., 1997; Kennedy et al., 2000).

Coban

Coban is a cohesive bandage that is commonly used by hand physiotherapists to aid the resolution of oedema, to improve scar tissue, prevent joint contracture and relieve pain (Boscheinen-Morrin and Conolly, 2001). Ward et al. (1994a) investigated the use of Coban wrap for management of post-burn hand grafts. It was found that the advantages of Coban were as follows:

- was self-adherent
- did not loosen
- fitted well
- was non-adherent to underlying tissues
- protected new grafts
- decreased oedema
- permited earlier mobility
- facilitated accurate measurement for pressure garments.

Once the grafts had become adherent and vascularized they were deemed suitable for the application of Coban and, even if dressings were still required, it could be used directly over them (Ward et al., 1994a). Coban can also be used to maintain a passively manipulated joint position.

Precautions when using compression:

- Whichever method of compression is chosen, and for whatever purpose, the main consideration must be the risk of compromising the circulation to the digit or hand. By leaving the tips of the digits exposed, the circulation can be monitored.
- Range of motion should not be restricted by the use of compressive dressings or garments (Sorenson, 1989).
- Compression is contraindicated if infection is present within the tissues (Sorenson, 1989; Palmada et al., 1999).

Silicone

Although Quinn (1987) demonstrated that the use of silicone on hypertrophic scarring was beneficial, the mechanism of how silicone improves the scar is unknown. Azad et al. (2000) described a number of theories:

- pressure, the compression afforded by the application of the silicone, is responsible for the improvement in the scar
- increased temperature
- reduced oxygen
- chemical effects
- increased hydration.

It is thought that the occlusive and hydration properties afforded by silicone provide the mode of action (Gollup, 2002). Baum and Busuito (1998) demonstrated this by achieving similar scarring results when they compared silicone with a glycerine-based sheet. Azad et al. (2000) noted that the use of silicone should be commenced as soon as a wound has healed and needs to be maintained for 12 hours a day for at least 2–4 months. However, Perkins et al. (1982) reported that silicone could be used to improve scarring for up to 12 months after healing. Despite this, Gollup (1988) reported that silicone was less beneficial on mature scars.

Van den Kerckhove et al. (2001) reported the methods of silicone application as follows:

- *Silicone fluids:* the hand is immersed in silicone fluid to facilitate wound healing and range of motion (Helal et al., 1982).
- *Silicone gel sheets:* these are applied directly over the scar and can either be used independently or beneath pressure garments.
- *Silicone elastomers:* tailormade silicone putty is placed under pressure garments or splints to fill concavities.
- *Silicone gels* (in tube): this is useful for areas of the body where it is difficult to apply gel sheets, such as the face.

Further reading

Van den Kerckhove E, Stappaerts K, Boeckx W, Van den Hot B, Monstrey S, Van der Kelen A et al. (2001) Silicones in the rehabilitation of burns: a review and overview. Burns 27: 205-14.

Splintage

Principles of splinting

To splint a joint effectively physiotherapists must understand its biomechanics (Colditz, 2000). All splints should have three points at which force is applied (Colditz, 2000). The central point should be over the joint that is to be affected; the other two points should be either side of the joint, as far away from the central point as is possible without affecting other joints (Colditz, 2000). The direction of force at the central point is opposite to the other two points. This principle can be used to immobilize or mobilize a joint (Colditz, 2000).

Physiology of splinting

One of the main uses of splintage is to regain range of joint motion by stretching soft tissues. There is still controversy over how elongation of tissue occurs during wound healing and splintage, that is, through stretching the tissues (Kottke et al., 1966) or the synthesis of new tissue (McClure et al., 1994). Most researchers agree that prolonged application of gentle, controlled stress results in the creation of new tissue and orientation of the collagen along the line of the stress, but definitive research is still lacking (Fess and McCollum, 1998).

Flowers and LaStayo (1994) found that the amount of transient versus permanent change in length of tissue was dependent upon the intensity and duration of the load applied. The longer a joint was positioned at end of range the greater the gain in passive range of motion. McClure et al. (1994) and Cyr and Ross (1998) also demonstrated that optimal plastic deformation occurred over a long period of low load stress.

The aims of splintage are as follows:

- pain relief and support to healing tissues during inflammation (Ashe, 2001)
- increase joint range of motion (Otthiers, 1998)
- restrict joint motion (Otthiers, 1998)
- maintain newly achieved joint range of motion (Palmada et al., 1999)
- maintain passive joint range of motion (Duncan, 1989)
- facilitate motion in one joint by positioning another joint (Duncan, 1989)
- protect joint integrity (Duncan, 1989)
- correct joint alignment (Duncan, 1989)
- support lax joints (Duncan, 1989)
- prevent deformity (Ranelli et al., 2000)
- protect tendon or nerve repairs (Irwin, 1999)
- prevent or correct contractures (Duncan, 1989)
- assist functional use of the hand (Leong, 1997)
- improve cosmesis (Azad et al., 2000)
- aid psychological recovery (Leong, 1997) by assisting function or independence.

Dynamic splints also aim to facilitate motion by:

- providing resistance
- providing prolonged stretch
- providing a substitution for weak or absent muscles or tendons (Duncan, 1989).

Categories of splintage

Splints can be either:

- static or dynamic
- supportive or corrective
- rigid or soft
- dorsal or volar
- digit-, hand- or forearm-based (Boscheinen-Morrin and Conolly, 2001).

The position of splintage depends on the position of safe immobilization of the hand (*see* Chapter 7) and the structures damaged. For example, after repair of the flexor tendons, the position of joint immobilization must not only prevent joint contractures but also protect the repaired tendons from being overstretched. Savage (1988) recommended that the least tensile demands on flexor tendon repairs were created with the wrist in slight flexion and metacarpophalangeal joints at 90° of flexion.

Splintage after burns

Splintage is not routinely necessary for burn-injured patients (Schnebly et al., 1989). If wounds and scars are monitored adequately for signs of deterioration, and if patients follow a rehabilitative regime that maintains range of motion, splints will only rarely be necessary. This protocol of appropriate rather than routine use prevents dependence on splinting devices and promotes patient independence (Schnebly et al., 1989). Despite this, some authors still recommend prophylactic splintage for particular areas of difficulty, for example the fifth metacarpophalangeal joint (Kennedy et al., 1998), to prevent complications such as anticipated contractures. The main purpose of splintage after burn injuries is to prevent contractures as the skin heals (*see* Chapter 6), and splints can be worn over pressure garments or silicone gel (Gollup, 2002).

Compliance with splintage

If patients find their splints relatively comfortable, they are more likely to comply with their use. To ensure compliance patients must understand the purpose of their splints. If possible, splints should be limited to night-time use to allow functional activity during the day; this is obviously not possible when splints are being used after surgery to protect reconstructed tissue. It may be fair to expect that custom-made splints fit better and are more useful or acceptable to patients. However, ter Schegget and Knipping (2000) found that prefabricated anti-swan neck splints were more tolerable to patients than tailor-made ones. To increase compliance with splint usage, especially with children, van Veldhoven, (2000) suggested using creative ideas for splints, for example aesthetically pleasing, decorative and fun designs.

Splinting precautions include the following:

- Precautions should be taken to ensure that splints do not produce friction or excessive pressure (Duncan, 1989) that could cause trauma to the soft tissues. Leong (1997) noted that there is a particular risk of pressure injury to skin after nerve injuries because of skin anaesthesia. Ranelli et al (2000) discussed the use of splintage after reconstructive surgery and noted the importance of avoiding pressure over the sites of anastomoses to prevent any compromise of circulation.
- Care should be taken when splinting children as small detachable pieces could be swallowed (Beresford, 1999). Beresford (1999) also noted that tape should be used to secure the splints on children rather than pins.
- The unnecessary use of splinting may cause venous and lymphatic stasis, which would result in an increase in oedema (Palmada et al., 1999).
- Splints need to be cleaned regularly to prevent colonization by microbes that could cause wound infection (Wright et al., 1989; Faoagali et al., 1994).
- A questionnaire by Mason (1992) elicited concern from surgeons over the skill of physiotherapists in splint making techniques, noting that an inexperienced splint maker could be potentially detrimental to patients' recovery. Weeks and Wray (1973) recommended that between 100 g and 300 g of force should be applied to finger joints and that the lighter forces within this range should be used for acute injuries and wounds. However, these authors demonstrated that inexperienced physiotherapists tended to select forces of more than 300 g and that this application of too much force caused microscopic tearing, oedema, inflammation and tissue necrosis. Hepburn (1987) also identified that the application of a high force for a short duration created an elastic response resulting in less remodelling, pain, weakening and possible rupture. These studies

seemed to substantiate the concerns expressed by surgeons in the survey by Mason (1992).

- Splintage should not be used in isolation but as part of a whole treatment plan (Leong, 1997).

Further reading

Duncan RM (1989) Basic principles of splinting the hand. Physical Therapy 69(11): 1104-16.

Thermal modalities

The use of heat or cold aims to relieve pain, reduce oedema and promote circulation in the area that is treated (McDowell et al., 1994). However, in acute injuries, the application of heat may increase oedema (Sorenson, 1989) and the application of ice will cause vasodilation that can also exacerbate inflammation (Salter and Bexon, 2000).

In the later stages of healing, heat reduces pain and facilitates active exercise, thereby aiding the resolution of swelling (Otthiers, 1998; Palmada et al., 1999). Palmada et al. (1999) also encouraged the use of heat in association with elevation to reduce pain, increase range of motion and reduce oedema, and they reported that the use of ice to cool the tissues would also result in an analgesic effect.

The application of heat to the hand is normally via a heat pack or a wax bath. The application of cold is via ice packs or ice water immersion. A number of devices are available to provide thermal therapy. Culp and Taras (1995) compared the use of ice packs with a cooling blanket on hands after surgery and concluded that the cooling blanket was more effective at cooling the tissues.

Contrast baths

The alternate immersion of the hand into warm then cool water will improve the circulation within the hand by improving the collateral blood supply (Salter and Bexon, 2000). This will result in resolution of oedema and reduced pain, which will facilitate motion and resumption of function.

Precautions

Great care must be taken in the application of thermal modalities, as there is the potential for tissue damage from heat or ice burns. Patients' sensation to heat and cold should be tested before their use. The application of thermal treatments is contraindicated over areas of anaesthetic skin because of the risk of tissue trauma.

Electrotherapy

Ultrasound

The most commonly used modality of electrotherapy is ultrasound (Pope et al., 1995); however, evidence for its effectiveness remains limited. The aim of ultrasound is to enhance the efficiency of the tissues natural healing process. Ward et al. (1994b) investigated the use of ultrasound on scarring and found that it did not produce any differences in range of motion or perceived pain when applied to burns patients. Cambier and Vanderstraeten (1997) also investigated the use of ultrasound in burn injuries with an aim of encouraging tissue healing, however, no significant effects were demonstrated.

There is limited research into the effects of ultrasound on tendon healing in human subjects (Rodger, 2000). Roberts et al. (1982) recommended that after tendon repairs the use of ultrasound should be delayed for 5 weeks because of its adverse effects on tendon healing. However, Gan et al. (1995) studied the effects of ultrasound on tendon repairs in chickens and claimed that the inclusion of ultrasound increased range of motion, advanced scar tissue maturation, decreased inflammatory infiltrate and had no adverse effects on tensile strength of the healed tendon. In previous studies by Enwemeka and Rodriguez (1990) and Jackson et al. (1991), the tensile strength of repaired tendons was shown to increase with the application of low-intensity ultrasound.

Transcutaneous electrical nerve stimulation (TENS)

Transcutaneous electrical nerve stimulation (TENS) utilizes natural pain relief mechanisms to provide analgesia. The pain gate mechanism (Melzack and Wall, 1965) reduces the transmission of the pain signals at the level of the spinal cord and the opioid mechanism causes the release of the body's own opiates, for example encephalins, which reduce the sensitivity of the sensory pathways.

An electrical stimulus is applied to the skin's sensory afferent fibres via electrodes. This application of the electrical current should be administered for 30–60 minutes (Boscheinen-Morrin and Conolly, 2001).

However, the nerves will gradually accommodate to the stimulus and it needs to be increased to continue to be effective.

Quinton et al. (1987) used TENS to modulate hand pain after infection and demonstrated that less analgesia was required and a greater range of motion achieved in those subjects who received TENS in the first 3 days post-operatively. Palmada et al (1999) reported that TENS aided reduction of oedema but the process of this reduction is not known although TENS does seem to increase the lymphatic uptake of proteins (Palmada et al., 1999).

Pulsed electromagnetic energy

The effects that are claimed to be attributable to pulsed electromagnetic energy are the restoration of normal cell membrane potential, the restoration of normal cell membrane transport mechanisms and therefore ionic balance. Goldin et al. (1981) stated that the aims of application of pulsed electromagnetic energy are to:

- increase the number of white blood cells, histocytes and fibroblasts
- reduce oedema (Barclay et al., 1983)
- stimulate re-absorption of haematoma
- reduce inflammation
- increase the rate of collagen deposition and scar orientation
- increase osteogenesis
- improve regeneration of nerves (Raji, 1984).

Neuromuscular electrical stimulation (NMES)

Neuromuscular electrical stimulation (NMES) can either be applied to innervated or denervated muscle. The potential beneficial effects of NMES are:

- pain relief
- improved local circulation
- reduction of oedema
- maintain joint range of motion
- maintain soft tissue glide
- modification of scar tissue or adhesions.

The application of an electrical stimulus to a denervated muscle via an electrode placed on the skin over a motor point within the muscle aims to produce a contraction within the muscle to retrain the muscle action and maintain tendon glide.

Muscle strengthening

The timing of inclusion of strengthening exercises depends on the structures that are damaged and their stage of healing. The gradual increase in strength of a muscle results from the progressive application of increased loads. This progression of treatment should be tailored to individual patients to be effective and prevent further injury or fatigue. Exercises aimed at increasing muscle power can be divided into strengthening exercises and endurance training, both of which are necessary for normal function.

Strengthening exercises

To increase the strength of a muscle it needs to be worked at a level close to its maximum capacity.

Endurance training

To increase the endurance of a muscle it needs to be worked at a reduced level of its maximum capacity for gradually increasing amounts of time. St-Pierre et al. (1998) noted that after severe burn injuries (>30% total body surface area) patients' muscle power remained reduced years after the injury. They suggested the cause was either inability to recover or insufficient rehabilitation. Roberts et al. (1993) also noted that grip strength remained lower than normative values 6 months after hand burn injury. However, despite this weakened grip, function was not necessarily a problem. Gripp et al. (1995) demonstrated the efficacy of a regime of muscle strengthening in burn-injured patients by developing a gymnasium at their burns unit to enable patients to continue with their rehabilitation independently.

Motor re-education

The resumption of motor function after nerve injury can be difficult because of atrophy of the muscle, the loss of normal patterns of motion and the adoption of trick movements. Ranelli et al. (2000) noted the need for motor re-education after tendon transfers to assist patients to learn the new action of transferred muscles.

Ranelli et al. (2000) recommended the use of functional activities to aid motor re-education, and Salter and Bexon (2000) suggested the following activities:

- isolated muscle activity
- application of a quick stretch to the muscle just before a contraction is attempted
- application of slight resistance in the direction of motion required to aid proprioception
- application of pressure over the muscle belly.

Sensory re-education

Anthony (1997) described the process of sensory re-education as 'a method by which the patient learns to interpret the pattern of abnormal sensory impulses generated after an interruption in the peripheral nervous system'. Salter and Bexon (2000) described the stages of nerve recovery by the sensations that patients feel:

- Initially, 'pins and needles' (hyperaesthesia) will be felt, this can be utilized as a protective sensation, that is, patients are able to identify heat or cold because of changes in hyperaesthesia.
- Next, patients will report shooting pains and will need reassuring that these sensations, though painful, are normal.
- The resolution of the pins and needles is replaced with a more normal but reduced sensation (hypoaesthesia).
- Gradually the hypoaesthesia progresses to a more normal sensation.

Sensory recovery is more rapid in children (Ranelli, 1998). Sensory re-education should be commenced when hypoaesthesia has been achieved in the hand (Anthony, 1997; Salter and Bexon, 2000).

The equipment used to re-educate sensation should be uncomplicated, readily available and cheap. With the vision occluded patients should first be encouraged to explore an object with the injured hand, and should attempt to describe it in terms of its size and texture. This exploration is aided or reinforced by the exploration of the object with the uninjured hand and visualization of the object (Ranelli, 1999; Salter and Bexon, 2000).

Localization of stimuli can also be improved with re-education. With the vision occluded a stimulus is applied to the area of reduced sensation, this stimulus may be moving or static, sharp or dull (Anthony, 1997). Patients can attempt to demonstrate where the sensation was perceived and describe its nature. Observation of the repeated application of the stimulus will reinforce the sensation.

Cold intolerance

Cold intolerance is worthy of a special mention as it is so frequently seen after any hand injury, particularly nerve injuries. Patients experience an exaggerated response to exposure of their hand to cold climates. Campbell and Kay (1998) described the symptoms as pain, numbness or tingling, stiffness and colour change. Rosen (1999) warned that it causes disuse and difficulty with activities of daily living.

The pathophysiology of cold intolerance is unknown but treatment includes education and advice about the avoidance of extreme temperatures and the use of gloves, self-heating bags, gel packs, battery powered gloves, etc. Irwin et al. (1997) reported factors that affected cold intolerance:

- age – worse in the elderly
- level of axonal recovery
- vascularity
- type of injury – worse in crushing injuries.

Desensitization

After hand trauma or surgery patients frequently experience hypersensitivity. Hypersensitivity is an 'exaggerated, painful response to a normally non-painful stimuli' (Anthony, 1997). Desensitization is the input of normal sensory stimuli to modulate the pain stimulus (Salter and Bexon, 2000).

Desensitization is most commonly needed after nerve injuries but it is also useful after any trauma that leaves extensive scarring, for example burn injuries (Clarke et al., 1997), and in the treatment of phantom sensations following amputation (Ranelli et al., 2000). To desensitize a hypersensitive area effectively patients' tolerance of the application of sensory stimuli is gradually increased (Anthony, 1997). Sensory stimuli, including vibration, a variety of textures, immersion in particles and pressure, are applied to the area of hypersensitivity in order of discomfort. For example, a selection of textures is applied to the area and patients grade them as 'bearable', 'unpleasant' and 'almost intolerable'. The textures are then applied to the area of hypersensitivity for a period of 5 minutes, in order from the most bearable to the almost intolerable. This activity is then repeated four to six times a day. As the hypersensitivity improves, new more irritating textures will need to be included.

Entonox

Pain can be a major limiting factor in the treatment of hand-injured patients. As has already been discussed, the normal movement patterns of the hand can be lost quickly (*see* Chapter 7) and active motion will prevent this loss. However, to enable patients to resume normal motion, pain must be controlled adequately (Collings, 1999). In order to control pain during treatment, therapy sessions should be timed around optimal analgesic periods. However, occasionally this is not practical and patients may require 'top-up' analgesia during treatment. Entonox is an ideal way of delivering a short-term analgesic with few side-effects. Entonox is a gas comprising 50% nitrous oxide and 50% oxygen. It is inhaled by patients via a self-administering system and is effective within a few breaths. It is excreted quickly via the respiratory system when patients remove the mouthpiece or mask.

Roe and Peck (1999) highlighted the advantages of Entonox:

- rapid onset
- rapid excretion
- low risk of overdose
- low risk of toxicity
- patients remain conscious and co-operative during treatment
- patient in control.

Roe and Peck (1999) also gave a comprehensive list of contraindications to the use of Entonox:

- chronic obstructive airways disease
- emphysematous bullae
- pneumothorax
- pneumoperitoneum
- head injuries
- inability to co-operate
- maxillofacial injuries
- unconsciousness
- heavy sedation
- intoxication
- air embolism
- decompression sickness
- recent underwater dive
- air encepalography
- myringoplasty
- bowel obstruction.

The presence of nausea or the risk of aspiration of vomit can be added to this list.

Acupuncture

Physiotherapists who wish to utilize acupuncture must first complete a postgraduate training course. For acupuncture to be effective, patients should experience a dull aching sensation around the needle (deqi). This stimulus is then transported to the central nervous system where it aids the blockage of the pain pathways (pain gate) or endorphins are released (Ellis, 1994). However, acupuncture will not treat the cause of the symptoms it will simply modulate the pain. It is particularly useful in the treatment of complex regional pain syndrome in association with other treatment modalities (Baker and Collings, 1997).

Psychological support

The importance of the hand to psychological well-being is immense. Although the main purpose of the hand is its use as a functional tool, it is also involved in communication, to express emotions or personality and to achieve contact with others and the world. The hand and its aesthetics are a very important part of creating body image.

After any injury, and sometimes after elective procedures (Cooper, 2001), patients will display signs of psychological disturbance as they struggle to come to terms with the injury or surgery and develop coping strategies. Pre-operative assessment of psychological status may be necessary for large elective procedures (Ranelli, 1998) and the parents of children undergoing surgery may need assistance.

Each patient is an individual and will react to situations differently. Physiotherapists should be able to identify when patients are developing psychological difficulties, help them to express their feelings, offer support where appropriate and know when referral to other professionals is necessary (Nichols, 1984; Ranelli et al., 2000). Nichols (1984) developed a four-part model of care that is a useful framework for physiotherapists to work within. The first part is emotional care: physiotherapists should demonstrate empathy and understanding by listening and encouraging patients to verbalize their feelings. Next is informational care: physiotherapists should give clear, accurate information in a manner that is acceptable to individual patients. Excellent communication skills are necessary to achieve this and the information given may need to be repeated on subsequent occasions until full understanding and acceptance is achieved. The third part of Nichol's (1984) model is basic counselling and the most important stage, monitoring or referral on to professional psychological help, follows this.

Coping strategies that may be employed by patients as they progress towards acceptance are:

- denial
- withdrawal
- drugs
- attention-seeking behaviour
- humour
- anger.

The best way to assist patients towards acceptance of their injury is to communicate openly. Patients needs time to grieve and should be reassured that it is all right to do so. A team approach to patient care will facilitate acceptance (*see* Chapter 5) and all members of the team need to give realistic and honest information to patients. The outcome of a hand injury depends on patients' personality and psychological state (Brand, 1996) so if physiotherapists can provide psychological support they will aid resolution of the physical problems too.

The close relationship that develops between physiotherapists and patients helps patients to accept their injury (Moore, 1999). Methods employed by physiotherapists to provide psychological support for patients are:

- education
- realistic encouragement and support
- holistic treatment
- individual treatment programmes
- achievable goal-setting (Moore, 1999).

Azad et al. (2000) noted the particular benefits of massage to aid acceptance of scarring. Nuse Pratt and Allen (1989) reported the importance of using functionally based activities and exercises with goal-orientated tasks to increase motivation and enhance self-esteem. Functional activities aid the restoration of confidence in the use of the hand and group sessions may aid social reintegration. Accepting responsibility for their own rehabilitation and recovery will give patients a greater sense of motivation and accomplishment (Gripp et al., 1995).

Functional activities

The use of functional activities to achieve desired results, for example increased range of joint motion and grip strength, forms the basis of occupational therapy. The utilization of functional activities and the sense of accomplishment as patients regain function is motivating to both patients and physiotherapists.

Functional activities aid the restoration of co-ordination of the hand. In the acute stages of treatment, physiotherapists concentrate on the restoration of the vital elements of function – joint range of motion, sensation, etc. However, in the later stages of treatment the inclusion of functional tasks helps patients to utilize their re-learnt skills by bringing them all together and re-learning normal patterns of movement.

Including functional activities in therapy sessions allows patients to practise activities in a 'safe' environment where they are not scrutinized by others. The opportunity to attend occupational therapy workshops also aids social re-integration and offers a chance for patients to regain confidence in the use of machinery. Occupational therapists can also supply a multitude of aids and adaptations to facilitate the use of everyday equipment. The level of functional activities included in treatment programmes should be progressive, as failure to achieve an activity can be demotivating.

Conclusion

There are numerous treatment modalities available for use by hand physiotherapists. The secret is to select the most appropriate modality, often this is done through experience and logic but if not it is advisable to select one modality at a time in order to evaluate its effect and not to become confused!

References

Angeras M, Brandberg A, Falk A, Seeman T (1992) Comparison between sterile saline and tap water for the cleaning of acute traumatic soft tissue wounds. European Journal of Surgery 158: 347-50.

Anthony MS (1997) Desensitisation. In: GL Clarke, EF Shaw Wilgis, B Aiello, D Eckhaus, L Valdata Eddington (eds). Hand Rehabilitation: A Practical Guide (second edition). London: Churchill Livingstone.

Appleby M (1997) The use of pressure garments in scar control. British Journal of Hand Therapy 2(6): 11-12.

Ashe MC (2001) Management of carpal instability: a therapist's perspective. British Journal of Hand Therapy 6(1): 9-14.

Azad SM, Gerrish J, Dziewulski P (2000) Hypertrophic scars and keloids: an overview of the aetiology and management. British Journal of Hand Therapy 5(1); 16-20.

Azad SM, Cherian A, Raine C, Dixon JE, Irvine BE, Erdmann MWH (2001) Dupuytren's disease: an overview of aetiology, pathology and treatment. British Journal of Hand Therapy 6(3): 73-8.

Baker A, Collings J (1997) Acupuncture and activity in the treatment of RSD. British Journal of Hand Therapy 2(6): 17-18.

Barclay V, Collier RJ, Jones A (1983) Treatment of various hand injuries by pulsed electromagnetic energy (diapulse). Physiotherapy 69(6): 186-8.

Barillo DJ, Harvey KD, Hobbs CL, Mozingo DW, Cioffi WG, Pruitt BA (1997) Prospective outcome analysis of a protocol for the surgical and rehabilitative management of burns to the hands. Plastic and Reconstructive Surgery 100(6): 1442-51.

Baum TM, Busuito MJ (1998) Use of a glycerine based gel sheeting in scar management. Advances in Wound Care 11: 40-3.

Beresford K (1999) Congenital hand anomaly: general considerations of care and management. British Journal of Hand Therapy 4(3): 112-18.

Boscheinen-Morrin J, Connolly WB (2001) The Hand: Fundamentals of Therapy. Oxford: Butterworth-Heinemann.

Brand PW (1996) Body and soul. Journal of Hand Therapy 9: 201-2.

Cambier DC, Vanderstraeten GG (1997) Failure of therapeutic ultrasound in healing burn injuries. Burns 23(3): 248-9.

Campbell DA, Kay SP (1998) What is cold intolerance? Journal of Hand Surgery 23B(1): 3-5.

Chang P, Laubenthal KM, Lewis RW, Rosenquist MD, Lindley-Smith P, Kealey GP (1995) Prospective randomised study of the efficacy of pressure garment therapy in patients with burns. Journal of Burn Care and Rehabilitation 16(5): 473-5.

Chester R, Davies J (2001) Combining passive movements to treat wrist joint dysfunction: a practical guide. British Journal of Hand Therapy 6(1): 21-5.

Clarke GL, Shaw Wilgis EF, Aiello B, Eckhaus D, Valdata Eddington L (1997) Hand Rehabilitation: A Practical Guide (second edition). London: Churchill Livingstone.

Colditz JC (2000) Efficient mechanics of proximal interphalangeal mobilization splinting. British Journal of Hand Therapy 5(3): 65-71.

Collings J (1999) The role of the fifth metacarpophalangeal joint in the recovery of the burnt hand - is it great or small? British Journal of Hand Therapy 4(1): 33-8.

Cooper A (2001) The mechanism and effect of Dupuytren's contracture. British Journal of Hand Therapy 6(3): 84-8.

Covey MH, Dutcher K, Marvin JA, Heimbach DM (1988) Efficacy of continuous passive motion (CPM) devices with hand burns. Journal of Burn Care and Rehabilitation 9(4): 397-400.

Cullen KW, Tolhurst P, Lang D, Page RE (1989) Flexor tendon repair in zone 2 followed by controlled active mobilization. Journal of Hand Surgery, 14B: 392-5.

Culp RW, Taras US (1995) The effect of ice application versus controlled cold therapy on skin temperature when used with postoperative bulky hand and wrist dressings: a preliminary study. Journal of Hand Therapy, 8(4): 249-51.

Cyr LM, Ross RG (1998) How controlled stress affects healing tissue. Journal of Hand Therapy, Apr-Jun: 125-30.

Duncan RM (1989) Basic principles of splinting the hand. Physical Therapy 69(11): 1104-16.

Ellis N (1994) Acupuncture in Clinical Practice - A Guide for Health Professionals. London: Chapman & Hall.

Enwemeka CS, Rodriguez O (1990) The biomechanical effects of low-intensity ultrasound on healing tendons. Ultrasound Med. Biol. 16(8): 801-7.

Faoagali JL, Grant D, Pegg S (1994) Are thermolabile splints a source of non-sociomial infection? Journal of Hospital Infection 26(1): 51-5.

Fess EE, McCollum M (1998) The influence of splinting on healing tissues. Journal of Hand Therapy, Apr–Jun: 157–61.

Field T, Peck M, Krugman S, Tuchel T, Schanberg S, Kuhn C et al. (1998) Burn injuries benefit from massage therapy. Journal of Burn Care and Rehabilitation 19(3): 241–4.

Flowers KR, LaStayo P (1994) Effects of total end range time on improving passive range of motion. Journal of Hand Therapy 3: 150–7.

Galley PM, Forster AL (1987) Human Movement. London: Churchill Livingstone.

Gan BS, Huys S, Sherebrin MH, Scilley CG (1995) The effects of ultrasound treatment on flexor tendon healing in the chicken limb. Journal of Hand Surgery 20B(6): 809–14.

Gelberman RH, Vandberg JS, Lundborg GN (1983) Flexor tendon healing, and restoration of the gliding surface: an ultrastructural study in dogs. Journal of Bone and Joint Surgery 65A: 70–80.

Goldin J, Broadbent NR, Nancarrow JD, Marshall T (1981) The effects of Diapulse on the healing of wounds: a double blind randomised controlled trial in man. British Journal of Plastic Surgery 34: 267–70.

Gollup R (1988) The use of silicone gel sheets in the control of hypertrophic scar tissue. British Journal of Occupational Therapy 51(7): 248–9.

Gollup R (2002) Burns aftercare and scar management. In: C Bosworth Bousfield. Burns Trauma, Management and Nursing Care (second edition). London: Whurr Publishers.

Gripp CL, Salvaggio J, Fratianne RB (1995) Use of burn intensive care unit gymnasium as an adjunct to therapy. Journal of Burn Care and Rehabilitation 16: 160–1.

Groth GN, Wulf MB (1995) Compliance with hand rehabilitation: health beliefs and strategies. Journal of Hand Therapy 8(1): 18–22.

Hayakawa T, Hino M, Fuyamada H (1977) Prolyl hydroxylase activity in human normal skin and post burn scars. Clin Chem Acta 75: 137–42.

Hepburn GR (1987) Case studies: contracture and stiff joint management with Dynasplint. Journal of Orthopaedic and Sports Physical Therapy 18(10): 498–504.

Herndon DN (1996) Total Burn Care. London: WB Saunders.

Hildebrand KA, Frank CB (1998) Scar formation and ligament healing. Canadian Journal of Surgery 41(6): 425–9.

Ip WY, Chow SP (1997) Results of dynamic splintage following extensor tendon repair. Journal of Hand Surgery 22B(2): 283–7.

Irwin MS (1999) Nerve repair and regeneration. British Journal of Hand Therapy 4(1): 8–12.

Irwin MS, Gilbert SEA, Terenghi G, Smith RW, Green CJ (1997) Cold intolerance following a peripheral nerve injury. Journal of Hand Surgery 22B(3): 308–16.

Jackson BA, Schwane JA et al. (1991) Effect of ultrasound therapy on the repair of Achilles tendon injury in rats. Medicine and Science in Sports and Exercise 23(2): 171–6.

Jefferis J, Dickinson J (1998) A joint approach in the treatment of an upper limb flexor division. British Journal of Hand Therapy 3(1): 5–6.

Jenkins M (1986) Failure of topical steroids and vitamin E to reduce post operative scar formation following reconstructive surgery. Journal of Burn Care and Rehabilitation 7(4): 309.

Kennedy S, Peck F, Stone J (1998) Prophylactic splintage of the 5th metacarpophalangeal joint in dorsal hand burns. British Journal of Hand Therapy 3(4): 22–3.

Kennedy S, Peck F, Stone J (2000) The treatment of interphalangeal joint flexion contractures with reinforced lycra finger sleeves. British Journal of Hand Therapy 5(2): 46–8.

Kottke FJ, Pauley DL, Ptak RA (1966) The rationale for prolonged stretching for correction of shortening connective tissue. Archives of Physical Medical Rehabilitation 47: 354–52.

Landsmeer J (1974) An Introduction to Functional Analysis of the Finger and Hand; Tendon Surgery of the Hand. St Louis, MI: CV Mosby.

Leong A (1997) The importance of splintage following a brachial plexus injury. British Journal of Hand Therapy 2(7): 10–12.

Maitland GD (1991) Peripheral Manipulation. London: Butterworth-Heinmann.

Mann R, Yeong EK, Moore M, Colescott D, Engrav LH (1997) Do custom-fitted pressure garments provide adequate pressure? Journal of Burn Care and Rehabilitation 18(3): 247-9.

Mason R (1992) The role of splintage in the post operative management of Dupuytren's contracture. British Journal of Hand Therapy 1(4): 6-12.

McClure PW, Blackburn LG, Dusold C (1994) The use of splints in the treatment of joint stiffness: biologic rationale and algorithm for making clinical decisions. Physical Therapy 74: 1101-7.

McDowell JH, McFarland EG, Malli BJ (1994) Use of cryotherapy for orthopaedic patients. Orthopaedic Nursing 13(5): 21-30.

Melzack R, Wall PD (1965) Pain mechanisms: a new theory. Science 150: 971-8.

Moore C (1999) A literature review into the psychological effects of traumatic hand injury and its implications for therapy. British Journal of Hand Therapy 4(3): 122-5.

Nichols K (1984) Psychological Care in Physical Illness. London: Croom Helm.

Nuse Pratt P, Allen AS (1989) Occupational Therapy for Children (second edition). St Louis, MI: CV Mosby.

Oliver L (1997) Wound cleansing. Nursing Standard 11(20): 47-56.

Otthiers J (1998) Rehabilitation of ligamentous injuries of the wrist. British Journal of Hand Therapy 3(3): 6-7.

Palmada M, Shah S, O'Hare K (1999) Hand oedema: pathophysiology and treatment. British Journal of Hand Therapy 4(1): 26-32.

Parsley C (1998) The progression of reflex sympathetic dystrophy and the implications for therapy. British Journal of Hand Therapy 3(1): 14-16.

Patino O, Novick C, Merlo A, Benaim F (1999) Massage in hypertrophic scars. Journal of Burn Care and Rehabilitation 20(3): 268-71.

Perkins K, Davey RB, Wallis KA (1982) Silicone gel: a new treatment for burn scars and contractures. Burns 9: 201-4.

Pope GD, Mockett S, Wright JP (1995) A survey of electrotherapeutic modalities: ownership and use in the NHS in England. Physiotherapy 81(2): 82-91.

Quinn KJ (1987) Silicone gel in scar treatment. Burns 13: 533-40.

Quinton DN, Sloan JP, Theakstone J (1987) Transcutaneous electrical nerve stimulation in acute hand infections. Journal of Hand Surgery 12-B(2): 267-8.

Raji AM (1984) An experimental study of the effects of pulsed electromagnetic field (diapulse) on nerve repair. Journal of Hand Surgery 9B(2): 105-12.

Ranelli S (1998) Controlled active extension programme in association with dynamic splinting for extensor tendon reconstruction zones three-eight. British Journal of Hand Therapy 3(1): 12-13.

Ranelli S, Forsythe S, Nanchahal J (2000) Principles of rehabilitation in reconstructive surgery in the upper limb. British Journal of Hand Therapy 5(1): 5-9.

Roberts M, Rutherford JH, Harris D (1982) The effect of ultrasound on flexor tendon repairs in the rabbit. The Hand 14(1): 17-20.

Roberts L, Alvarada MI, McElroy K, Rutan RL, Desai MH, Herndon DN et al. (1993) Longitudinal hand grip and pinch strength recovery in the child with burns. Journal of Burn Care and Rehabilitation 14(1): 99-101.

Rodger J (2000) The role of ultrasound in the treatment of surgically repaired tendon injuries of the hand: a literature review. British Journal of Hand Therapy 5(2): 42-5.

Roe A, Peck F (1999) Entonox - an effective analgesic for painful physiotherapy procedures. British Journal of Hand Therapy 4(2): 60-3.

Ronon C (2001) The use of massage to influence collagen synthesis in the hand: a physiological justification. British Journal of Hand Therapy 6(3): 95-9.

Rosen B (1999) Cold intolerance in the hand - an unsolved problem. British Journal of Hand Therapy 4(1): 23-5.

Salter RB (1996) History of rest and motion and the scientific basis of continuous passive motion. Hand Clinics 12(1): 1-11.

Salter M, Bexon C (2000) Treatment. In: M Salter, L Cheshire. Hand Therapy: Principles and Practice. Oxford: Butterworth-Heinemann.

Savage R (1988) The influence of wrist position on the minimum force required for active movement of the interphalangeal joints. Journal of Hand Surgery 13B: 262-8.

Schnebly WA, Ward RS, Warden GD, Saffle JR (1989) A non-splinting approach to the care of the thermally injured patient. Journal of Burn Care and Rehabilitation 10(3): 263-6.

Silverskjold K, May E, Tornvall A (1992) Flexor digitorum profundus tendon excursions during controlled motion after flexor tendon repair in zone two: a prospective clinical study. Journal of Hand Surgery 17A: 122-31.

Simons P, Coleridge Smith P, Lees WR, McGrowther DA (1996) Venous pumps of the hand: their clinical importance. Journal of Hand Surgery 21B: 595-9.

Small J, Brennen M, Colville J (1989) Early active mobilization following flexor tendon repair in zone 2. Journal of Hand Surgery 14B: 383-91.

Sorenson MK (1989) The edematous hand. Physical Therapy 69(12): 1059-64.

Staley MJ, Richard RL (1997) Use of pressure to treat hypertrophic burn scars. Advances in Wound Care 10(3): 44-6.

St Pierre DM, Choiniere M, Forget R, Garrel DR (1998) Muscle strength in individuals with healed burns. Archives of Physical Medicine and Rehabilitation 79(2): 155-61.

ter Schegget M, Knipping A (2000) A study comparing use and effects of custom made versus prefabricated splints for swan neck deformity in patients with rheumatoid arthritis. British Journal of Hand Therapy 5(4): 101-7.

Thompson R, Summers S, Rampey-Dobbs R, Wheeler T (1992) Colour pressure garments versus traditional beige pressure garments: perceptions from the public. Journal of Burn Care and Rehabilitation 13: 590-6.

Van den Kerckhove E, Stappaerts K, Boeckx W, Van den Hof B, Monstrey S, Van der Kelen A et al. (2001) Silicones in the rehabilitation of burns: a review and overview. Burns 27: 205-14.

Van Veldhoven G (2000) Creativity in splinting. British Journal of Hand Therapy 5(3): 77-9.

Ward RS (1991) Pressure therapy for the control of hypertrophic scar formation after burn injury. Journal of Burn Care and Rehabilitation 12: 257-62.

Ward RS, Reddy R, Brockway C, Hayes-Lundy C, Mills P (1994a) Uses of Coban self adherent wrap in management of post-burn hand grafts: case reports. Journal of Burn Care and Rehabilitation 15(4): 364-9.

Ward RS, Hayes-Lundy C, Reddy R, Brockway C, Mills P, Saffle JR (1994b) Evaluation of topical therapeutic ultrasound to improve response to physical therapy and lessen scar contracture after burn injury. Journal of Burn Care and Rehabilitation 15(1): 74-9.

Weeks PM, Wray RC (1973) Management of Acute Hand Injuries: A Biologic Approach. St Louis, MI: CV Mosby.

Williams P (1980) Gray's Anatomy (36th edition). London: Churchill Livingstone.

Wright MP, Taddonio TE, Prasad JK, Thomson PD (1989) The microbiology and cleaning of thermoplastic splints in burn care. Journal of Burn Care and Rehabilitation 10(1): 79-83.

Chapter 10

Case studies

Case study 1: Flexor tendon repair in zone 2

Demographic outline

A 36-year-old woman was referred with a laceration to her dominant right index finger. The injury was sustained on a broken cup. The laceration was small but deep, extending over the volar aspect of her proximal interphalangeal joint. On examination, she had reduced sensation in the fingertip and was unable to actively flex either of the interphalangeal joints.

The patient had no relevant previous medical history and did not take any regular medication. She was married with one 2-year-old child and worked part-time in a factory, where her job involved lifting boxes.

On surgical examination of the injury, it was found that both the flexor digitorum profundus and superficialis tendons had been divided, as had the radial digital nerve of the index finger. The proximal portions of the tendons had retracted into the palm, therefore the wound was extended proximally to facilitate their recovery. The tendons were repaired by use of a modified Kessler locking suture and an epitendinous suture; free gliding of the tendons beneath the pulleys was established before wound closure. The radial digital nerve was also repaired. Post-operatively a dorsal blocking plaster of Paris splint was applied and the patient was returned to the ward with the hand elevated. The operating surgeon and the specialist plastic surgery nurses warned the patient not to attempt any active motion in the hand until she was seen by the physiotherapist the next day.

Assessment

The patient was reviewed by the operating surgeon and the physiotherapist the day after surgery. The injury, operation and implications of rehabilitation were explained to her by both the surgeon and the physiotherapist. The patient was given time to understand the information and the opportunity to ask questions. The patient expressed shock and disbelief at the amount of rehabilitation that she would require and the amount of time that she would need away from work. Although she had been warned of the severity of the injury pre-operatively, she had still believed that once the wound had been sutured she would be able to return to her normal activities immediately. The patient did not appreciate the severity of the injury and needed time to accept it.

The hand dressings were removed and upon observation, the wound was found to be clean and intact. There was no evidence of excessive erythema, pus or pain, which could have been indicative of infection. As the wound was clean and dry, a light dressing was applied.

Once a thermoplastic dorsal blocking splint had been made and was in place on the patient's hand to protect the tendon repairs, the tendons could be tested for continuity and glide. The joint positions within the splint were:

- wrist neutral
- metacarpophalangeal joints at 70° flexion
- proximal interphalangeal and distal interphalangeal joints in extension.

To test the continuity of the flexor digitorum profundus tendon, the digit was gently supported just proximal to the distal interphalangeal joint in order to limit the action of the flexor digitorum superficialis tendon on the proximal interphalangeal joint. Active flexion of the distal interphalangeal joint proved that the flexor digitorum profundus tendon was intact and gliding. To test the continuity of the flexor digitorum superficialis tendon, the ulnar three digits were immobilized while the patient was asked to actively flex the index finger. By immobilizing the other three digits the flexor digitorum profundus tendons, which normally work together, would be immobilized. Therefore, active flexion of the proximal interphalangeal joint of the index finger was attributed to the intact flexor digitorum superficialis tendon.

As the compressive postoperative dressings had been removed, the digit was liable to swell. The extent of this oedema was recorded to give a baseline measurement with which subsequent assessments could be compared. To assess the oedema (*see* Chapter 8) the circumference of the digit was measured at mid-proximal phalanx and mid-middle phalanx levels. On the affected digit, both measurements were found to be 0.5 cm greater than the contralateral digit. A more accurate method of assessing hand oedema is the measurement of volumetric displacement (Boland and Adams, 1996) but this method was impractical for regular reassessment and the circumferential measurement method was deemed sufficient for clinical use.

The extent of sensory loss was assessed (*see* Chapter 8) using a dynamic two-point discrimination test (Dellon, 1978) and the results were documented on a sensory map of the hand to aid comparison at subsequent assessments. This sensory assessment tool was chosen, despite the opportunity for its application to be variable (Bell-Krotoski et al., 1993), as it is clinically quick to use and is appropriate to test fingertip sensation (Bell-Krotoski et al., 1993). Assessment of the index finger revealed that the two points could be correctly identified on the ulnar side of the digit at a distance of 3 mm apart. However, on the radial aspect of the finger the patient was unable to correctly identify the difference between the application of two points and one point.

Because of the nature of the injury, the patient would not be able to use the hand functionally for 6 weeks (Boardman and Salter, 2000). Therefore, the evaluation of hand function was limited to establishing the patient's functional requirements for her personal and professional life. This discussion would be useful in setting goals and treatment planning. The patient's initial concern was how she would manage the care of her 2-year-old son. Fortunately, the patient was entitled to paid sick leave from her job, therefore financial worries would not be an issue during rehabilitation. The only hobby that the patient reported that involved the use of her hands was reading.

Problems identified and priorities

After the initial assessment the problems identified were:

- lack of knowledge and understanding of the injury and its implications
- wound management
- risk of reduced range of joint motion
- oedema
- reduced sensation
- educed grip strength
- loss of hand function.

The initial priority was the patient's lack of knowledge and understanding of the injury, the surgery and the implications of the rehabilitation process. If patients can understand their injuries and the reasons why they must follow a strict rehabilitation regime, they are more likely to comply with their treatment (Groth and Wulf, 1995).

A wound infection would have been disastrous to the recovery of this patient. The patient would require bulky dressings and topical treatments to resolve the infection, which could have precluded the application of an appropriate exercise regime (Small et al., 1989). Infection could also have prolonged the inflammatory phase of tissue healing, delaying the healing process and exacerbating the development of scar tissue that would cause adhesions within the flexor sheath and reduce tendon glide (Wilson, 1983). Every effort was made, therefore, to prevent infection by ensuring the wound was kept clean and dry, and was monitored regularly.

Once flexor tendons have been repaired, their mobility must be maintained to ensure that the inevitable scar tissue does not cause them to adhere to the walls of the flexor sheath and to each other (Peck et al., 1998). However, whilst maintaining this tendon glide with active motion it is important not to place excessive strain through the delicate repairs as this could cause repair lengthening or even rupture (Elliot et al., 1994). A strictly controlled exercise regime was necessary to maintain tendon glide yet protect the repairs (Gelberman et al., 1986).

Excessive oedema can cause a reduction in the ability to mobilize the joints of the hand (Palmada et al., 1999). The importance of maintaining tendon excursion has already been established and if excessive oedema was allowed to persist this could cause joint stiffness, leading to undue resistance to the contraction of the flexors of the digits. Reducing oedema ensures that unresisted tendon excursion is maintained. This tendon motion facilitates continuous 'milking' of synovial fluid within the sheath, which provides the healing tendons with the majority of their nutrition. Oedema within a digit can potentially cause a reduction in tissue perfusion because of an increase in pressure, leading to compression of the smaller blood vessels (Trofino, 1991). As there was evidence that the vinculae had been damaged in this patient, due to the unopposed retraction of the proximal portions of the severed tendons at the time of surgery, digital circulation had to be preserved to create the best environment for wound, tendon and nerve healing.

Even though the digital nerve had been repaired, the resolution of sensation would not be expected for a number of months. The priority was to explain the process of nerve degeneration and regeneration to the patient, to reassure her and to educate her about skin care and the protection of the anaesthetic skin to ensure that she did not suffer any further injuries.

Maintenance of grip strength was a low priority at this early stage of tendon repair as any resisted exercise that was designed to strengthen the musculature of the hand and forearm would damage the delicate tendon repairs. Urbaniek et al. (1975) demonstrated that strong digital flexion, needed to improve grip strength, produced a force of 5 kg. Strickland and Glogovac (1980) showed that even a six-strand modified Kessler suture would only withstand 2.7 kg at 1 week and 3.6 kg at 3 weeks postoperatively.

Inevitably, the patient's priority was the resumption of hand function. Careful, consistent explanations regarding the importance of refraining from attempting to use the injured hand for the first 6 weeks were necessary.

Goals, aims and objectives

Setting agreed goals with the patient was an essential part of the treatment process. She was encouraged to take responsibility for her rehabilitation, and participating in setting achievable goals initiated this.

Aims and objectives were clearly defined and timed so that they could be reviewed. It was expected that this patient would achieve full understanding and knowledge of her injury and its implications after a month of rehabilitation. This may seem like a long time to gain insight into an injury but the patient required repeated explanations of the complex processes of tissue healing, scarring and the biomechanics of the injured hand. She also needed time to accept the injury and to build a rapport with the physiotherapist so that she felt confident enough to ask questions about her rehabilitation.

With correct management, this patient's wound should have been healed within 2 weeks. Once wound healing had been achieved, scar management techniques could be commenced.

After an uncomplicated repair of the flexor tendons at this level, it would be expected that patients should achieve full passive flexion and extension of all the digits within the dorsal blocking splint by 2–3 weeks after the operation. Virtually full active flexion and extension within the splint should also be achieved by 2 weeks after surgery (Peck et al., 1998). This active range of motion should continue to improve slowly until the full range of active flexion and extension of all the joints is achieved at between 8 and 12 weeks post-operatively (Peck et al., 1998).

With appropriate treatment, complete resolution of oedema should be achieved by 3 months after the injury. However, a period of fluctuation of oedema can be expected during this time.

The patient should gradually begin to notice the return of some sensations within the radial aspect of the digit after approximately 2 months, although these may be limited to generalized hyperaesthesia or paraesthesia (Boscheinen-Morrin and Conolly, 2001). Because of the slow axonal growth rate (of a maximum of 1 mm a day) and the misdirection of axons (Lundborg, 1999), complete recovery of sensation is unlikely, but the extent of recovery should be known by 6 months post-operatively, as the more distal the injury the better the prognosis of nerve recovery (Irwin, 1999).

The restoration of grip strength is addressed when tendon repairs are strong enough to withstand resisted exercise, that is, 12 weeks after surgery (Peck et al., 1998). Full grip strength should be achievable by 4–6 months after injury.

Because of the loss of sensation in the radial aspect of the index finger, the patient may initially not use the digit. Physiotherapy aims to educate patients about the cause of this non-use and to encourage the inclusion of the digit in functional activities in order to facilitate the resumption of full hand function. Full functional use of the hand should be available to patients 3–4 months post-operatively, despite the possible persistent loss of sensation.

Treatment programme

The patient's hand was placed in a thermoplastic dorsal blocking splint (*see* Chapter 9) for the first 6 weeks after surgery to protect the tendon repairs (Cullen et al., 1989). As discussed previously, a large proportion of initial treatment sessions consisted of patient education (*see* Chapter 9) about the nature of the injury and its implications, followed by the need for compliance with the treatment programme.

In order to maintain tendon glide within the flexor sheath during tendon healing, whilst preventing tendon rupture, the patient followed a controlled active motion regime (Small et al., 1989). This was a balance of rest and exercise that was specifically designed to achieve these objectives (Cullen et al., 1989). It has been demonstrated that early controlled motion after a flexor tendon repair increases the tensile strength of the repair (Gelberman and Woo, 1989). An example of this exercise regime is:

- two passive flexion and extensions to each digit individually
- two active flexion and extensions (all digits move together).

This combination of exercises was completed four times a day for the first 6 weeks (Cullen et al., 1989). On removal of the splint at 6 weeks, the exercises were increased in their frequency and included active extension of the metacarpophalangeal joints (Cullen et al., 1989). Had the patient developed a flexion contracture at the proximal interphalangeal joint a night extension splint would have been applied (Peck et al., 1998) and protected passive extension exercises commenced.

Oedema was addressed by elevating the limb at all times (Palmada et al., 1999). The application of a light compressive bandage also aided resolution of oedema (Salter and Cheshire, 2000).

Sensory recovery was monitored and once it had reached the fingertip a regime of sensory re-education (*see* Chapter 9) could be commenced to aid the patient to relearn the interpretation of sensory stimuli.

A programme of gradually increasing resisted exercises was initiated at 12 weeks post-operatively in order to aid the patient to regain full grip strength (*see* Chapter 9). The strength of both the intrinsic and extrinsic muscles of the hand needed to be addressed to achieve a balance of power for all types of grip.

Light hand function could begin as soon as the splint was removed at 6 weeks (Cullen et al., 1989). This was gradually upgraded until 12 weeks, when the tendons were deemed strong enough to withstand full function. Because of the loss of sensation in the index finger, the patient was at risk of not using the digit. This was strongly discouraged.

Progress report and alterations to regime

At 2 weeks post-operatively, the patient noted that the splint no longer felt comfortable. On examination it was found that the hand oedema had successfully been reduced by strict elevation; however, this had the effect of making the forearm part of the splint too large. The splint was altered to improve comfort and maintain compliance. In addition, at 2–3 weeks after surgery, the patient was encouraged to increase the effort of active flexion; this was because the tendon repairs had survived the most deli- cate inflammatory stage of tendon healing and had entered the proliferative stage of healing, where a level of controlled stretch would facilitate tendon healing and increase tensile strength (Strickland, 1989).

At 4 weeks post-operatively, there was a lack of active flexion within the digits. Therefore individual blocking exercises (*see* Chapter 9) for the finger joints were added to the regime to achieve differential gliding between the tendons, preventing intertendinous adhesions.

At 6 weeks, the dorsal blocking split was removed and exercise was increased in frequency, whilst light activities were commenced (Cullen et al., 1989). This treatment progress required a full explanation to the patient and she was reassured that the tendon repairs were now strong enough to withstand this activity. Initially, there was a lack of active metacarpophalangeal joint extension, however after a further 4 weeks' rehabilitation full range of all the joints was achieved except for a slight lack of index finger distal interphalangeal joint flexion. This was attrib- uted to adhesions around the flexor digitorum profundus tendon and was addressed with increased blocking exercises and scar massage (*see* Chapter 9). Joint range of motion was assessed (*see* Chapter 8) by use of goniometry (Boone et al., 1978).

At the time of discharge from physiotherapy, sensation in the radial aspect of the digit was limited to hyperaesthesia in the radial side of the fingertip. On examination, dynamic two-point discrimination was measured at 11 mm.

Hand function was gradually increased as the patient gained confidence. She was able to return to work on light duties at 10 weeks post-operatively, and gradually upgraded her function and grip strength until she was able to return to full function at 12 weeks (Peck et al., 1998). At this stage, the continued risks of anaesthetic skin were re-emphasized, and although the patient was discharged from physiotherapy, she would attend the consultant hand clinic to monitor her nerve recovery. If it was considered necessary to re-educate the patient once her sensation had returned to her fingertip, she would be re-referred to physiotherapy at that stage.

Summary

This case study demonstrates the uncomplicated rehabilitation of a patient after flexor tendon repair. The physiotherapist had to employ her/his skills in education and communication in order to establish a rapport with the patient. The balance of graded motion and rest was ensured to allow optimal tendon healing whilst maintaining tendon nutrition and glide. The gradual restoration of hand function was controlled to prevent any setbacks and potential complications, such as adhesions or non-use, were addressed before they became a problem. The patient's goal – to regain virtually complete range of motion and to resume all pre-injury activities – was achieved. Further physiotherapy may be necessary to teach sensory re-education at a later stage. For this lady, referral to other disciplines proved unnecessary. However, had the patient experienced difficulty in resumption of hand function or restoration of grip strength, occupational therapy would have been required. Fortunately, she did not experience any psychological effects after her injury; had this occurred a referral to the clinical psychologist would have been arranged. Because of the experience of the therapy team, the patient was only reviewed by the hand consultant at discharge from physiotherapy. If there had been any complications during the rehabilitative process or if the physiotherapist was not as experienced, a more regular medical review would have been arranged.

To achieve successful rehabilitation of a flexor tendon injury physiotherapists must use their skills and knowledge in education, anatomy, pathology, tissue healing and biomechanics to ensure optimal recovery is achieved.

References

Bell-Krotoski J, Weinstein S, Weinstein C (1993) Testing sensibility, including touch-presure, two-point discrimination, point localisation, and vibration. Journal of Hand Therapy Apr-Jun: 114-23.

Boardman S, Salter M (2000) Specific conditions and injuries. In: M Slater, L Cheshire (eds) Hand Therapy: Principles and Practice. Oxford: Butterworth-Heinemann.

Boland R, Adams R (1996) Development and evaluation of a precision forearm and hand volumeter and measuring cylinder. Journal of Hand Therapy 9(4): 349-58.

Boone DC, Azen SP, Lin CM (1978) Reliability of goniometric measurements. Physical Therapy 58: 1355-60.

Boscheinen-Morrin J, Connolly WB (2001) The Hand: Fundamentals of Therapy (third edition). Oxford: Butterworth-Heinemann.

Cullen KW, Tolhurst P, Lang D, Page RE (1989) Flexor tendon repair in zone 2 followed by controlled active mobilisation. Journal of Hand Surgery 14B: 392-5.

Dellon AL (1978) The moving two-point discrimination test: clinical evaluation of the quickly adapting fibre/receptor system. Journal of Hand Surgery 3: 474.

Elliot D, Moiemen NS, Flemming AFS, Harris SB, Foster AJ (1994) The rupture rate of acute flexor tendon repairs mobilised by the controlled active motion regimen. Journal of Hand Surgery 19B(5): 607-12.

Gelberman RH, Botte MJ, Spiegelman JJ, Akeson WH (1986) The excursion and deformation of repaired flexor tendons treated with protected early motion. Journal of Hand Surgery 11A: 106-10.

Gelberman RH, Woo SL-Y (1989) The physiological basis for the application of controlled stress in the rehabilitation of flexor tendon injuries. Journal of Hand Therapy 2: 66.

Groth GN, Wulf MB (1995) Compliance with hand rehabilitation: health beliefs and strategies. Journal of Hand Therapy 8(1): 18-22.

Irwin MS (1999) Nerve repair and regeneration. British Journal of Hand Therapy 4(1): 8-12.

Lundborg G (1999) Nerve repair: current concept and future prospectives. British Journal of Hand Therapy 4(1): 5-7.

Palmada M, Shah S, O'Hare K (1999) Hand oedema: pathophysioloy and treatment. British Journal of Hand Therapy 4(1): 26-32.

Peck FH, Bucher CA, Watson JS, Roe A (1998) A comparative study of two methods of controlled mobilisation of flexor tendon repairs in zone 2. Journal of Hand Surgery 23B(1): 41-5.

Salter M, Cheshire L (2000) Hand Therapy: Principles and Practice. Oxford: Butterworth-Heinemann.

Small J, Brennen M, Colville J (1989) Early active mobilisation following flexor tendon repair in zone 2. Journal of Hand Surgery 14B: 383-91.

Strickland JK, Glogovac SV (1980) Digital function following flexor tendon repair in zone 2: a comparison of immobilisation and controlled passive motion techniques. Journal of Hand Surgery (Am) 5: 537-43.

Strickland JW (1989) Biological rationale, clinical application, and results of early motion following flexor tendon repair. Journal of Hand Therapy Apr-Jun: 71-83.

Trofino RB (1991) Nursing Care of the Burn Injured Patient. Philadelphia, PA: FA Davies.

Urbaniek JR, Cahill JD, Mortensor RA (1975) Tendon suturing methods: analysis of tendon strengths. In: American Academy of Orthopedic Surgeons Symposium on Tendon Surgery in the Hand. St Louis, MI: CV Mosby; 70-80.

Wilson DH (1983) Tensynovitis, tenovaginitis and trigger finger. Physiotherapy 69(10): 350-2.

Case study 2: Physiotherapy after a fingertip amputation

Demographic outline

An 18-year-old lady sustained a traumatic partial amputation of the tip of her left, non-dominant, middle finger after it was caught in a door. The patient had no relevant history and was a student who lived with her parents and did not have any hand-based hobbies.

On attending the Accident and Emergency Department, it was decided that the fingertip was unsalvageable because of the level of amputation and the extent of the crushing trauma to the tissues (Boulas, 1998). The most appropriate option, therefore, was terminalization of the digit. The surgical intervention was performed by an Accident and Emergency doctor under local anaesthetic. Eventually, owing to a lack of recovery, the patient was referred for physiotherapy from the Accident and Emergency follow-up clinic, one and half months after the accident.

The decision to amputate this digit would not have been taken lightly. It is known that the loss of the middle finger represents a loss of 20% of hand function (Boscheinen-Morrin and Connolly, 2001). In addition, the length and central position of the middle finger facilitates its role in both activities that require precision and those that require strength (Boscheinen-Morrin and Connolly, 2001).

Assessment

Two months after the injury the patient attended physiotherapy. On initial examination, the patient was extremely distressed and traumatized by the accident, and her subsequent treatment. She described the procedure of terminalization of the digit as excruciatingly painful. She noted that she could feel and hear the doctor nibbling back the bone. Since the surgery, she had attended the Accident and Emergency clinic once and was unhappy with the consultation that she had received.

On palpation of the digit, it was severely hypersensitive. The patient was very reluctant to allow it to be touched and she had not washed it since the accident so the tip remained covered by old blood. The whole of her hand was oedematous and because of its appearance, the patient was self-conscious and was attempting to keep it covered. A baseline measurement of hand oedema was not taken owing to the patient's distress, but on subsequent physiotherapy sessions this was done using circumferential measurements (*see* Chapter 8). The range of motion in all the digits was reduced on goniometric examination (*see* Chapter 8) (Boone et al., 1978) and the patient was not using the hand.

Goals, aims and objectives

From the initial assessment the following priorities were established:

- gain trust and build rapport with the patient
- provide psychological support and refer to clinical psychologist as necessary
- educate and gain compliance
- desensitize the fingertip
- reduce oedema
- increase finger joint range of motion
- restore function with the aid of occupational therapy intervention.

Treatment

The treatment priority for this patient was to gain trust and to build rapport without dependency (Parsley, 1998). The first physiotherapy session consisted of explanations and reassurance. The hand was soaked in warm soapy water to lift the old blood and to demonstrate to the patient that the wound was healed. A stitch was found to be remaining in the wound but the patient was unable to tolerate its removal. The warmth of the water provided pain relief, improved skin condition and aided mobility of the hand (Otthiers, 1998). Gentle massage with moisturizing cream (*see* Chapter 9) was initiated to gain the patient's confidence in touching the digit (Cheshire, 2000) and to reduce her anxiety (Field et al., 1998), but care was taken not to increase the patient's pain, which would exacerbate her anxiety and mistrust. A full explanation of disuse and hypersensitivity was given, allowing the patient time to understand and ask questions. An exercise regime was devised with the patient's agreement.

Active exercise with the inclusion of isolated joint exercises (*see* Chapter 9) were commenced to reduce joint stiffness, regain tendon glide (Small et al., 1989) and to reduce oedema (Palmada et al., 1999). Passive movements (*see* Chapter 9) were also used to increase range of motion. A desensitization programme (*see* Chapter 9) was taught to normalize sensory input and modulate pain (Salter and Bexon, 2000). This treatment regime would have normally been initiated at 10–14 days after the injury (Boscheinen-Morrin and Connolly, 2001).

On subsequent visits to the physiotherapy department, the treatment programme was developed as the patient gained confidence. Most time was spent educating the patient and reassuring her that compliance with the activities would not be detrimental despite being uncomfortable. The patient was also advised to visit her general practitioner to review her analgesic requirements. Oedema was reduced by use of compression bandages (Sorenson, 1989), active exercise (Palmada et al., 1999) and retrograde massage (Sorenson, 1989). The hypersensitivity began to improve after the initiation of the desensitising programme. Eventually, 3 months after the injury, the patient was able to tolerate the removal of the residual stitch from the fingertip. Functional exercises (see Chapter 9) were introduced into the rehabilitation programme to address the continued non-use of the digit, and strengthening exercises were commenced. At this stage, the patient was referred to the occupational therapy department to enhance her functional recovery.

Re-assessment and modification of treatment

Five months after the injury the patient returned to the Accident and Emergency clinic. It became evident that she was becoming increasingly depressed by the continued discomfort she was experiencing in the digit. She was now complaining of metacarpophalangeal joint pain, which was attributed to the joint being held in hyperextension in order to avoid contact of the fingertip with objects that would cause pain. Despite her continued efforts to desensitize the digit and include it in functional activities the hypersensitivity seemed to plateau. It was at this point that the physiotherapist contacted the Accident and Emergency consultant and requested that the patient be referred to a specialist hand surgeon. The suspicion that the pain was being caused by the presence of a neuroma needed to be investigated.

The patient attended a joint hand consultant and physiotherapy clinic so that the physiotherapist could brief the surgeon on the history of the case and inform him of all the procedures and progress that the patient had made. The consultant agreed that there was evidence of a neuroma in the fingertip and was able to discuss the treatment options with the patient. The patient was extremely reluctant to have any further surgical intervention. However, because of the relationship that the physiotherapist had been able to build with the patient, and the physiotherapist's inclusion in the discussions with the surgeon, the patient agreed to the surgical option of excision of neuroma with nail ablation. It was decided that surgery would take place under general anaesthetic by the consultant himself, with a pre-arranged physiotherapy appointment on the day after surgery.

During the surgical refashioning of the finger stump the nail bed was ablated to prevent any further growth and two large neuromas were excised. On the day after surgery, the patient was initially very anxious but physiotherapy was commenced immediately and the patient noted an improvement in the sensitivity of the digit. The exercise programme was recommenced with the addition of Coban wrapping (*see* Chapter 9) to shape the stump, and the provision of a cosmetic prosthesis for use when required (Jones, 1997). On discharge from physiotherapy, 10 months after her original injury, the patient was able to use her hand fully and the sensation in the fingertip was continuing to improve.

Psychological response to amputation

It is clear from this case study that this lady's psychological well-being was severely affected by her injury. In an ideal situation the patient should have been assessed for the likely psychological impact that terminalization would have upon her and every effort should have been made to reassure and explain the situation to her. Most importantly, the surgical procedure should have been pain-free, as this experience further compounded the trauma that she had already suffered and led to fear and mistrust of the medical professionals that would later try to aid her recovery. A great deal of time needed to be taken winning the trust of this patient as it was only when this trust was gained that she had the courage to comply with her treatment programme (Cheshire, 2000). Each patient should be treated as an individual. A person may be traumatized more by the loss of one fingertip than another person who has lost multiple digits (Boscheinen-Morrin and Connolly, 2001). Cheshire (2000) emphasized this point in her comparison of the effect of the loss of a fingertip in a schoolteacher compared with a pianist. The evidence of this patient's non-use and hiding of the hand demonstrates the effect that this injury had on her body image and self-esteem (Boscheinen-Morrin and Connolly, 2001). Had the delay between injury and referral to physiotherapy been reduced, these effects could have been counteracted by education and emotional support. Often, patients with a small visible injury will not receive the psychological support that they need as the trauma is perceived by others to be minimal and insignificant (Cheshire, 2000). However, it is this attitude from friends, family and some inexperienced medical professionals that can enhance patients' distress (Cheshire, 2000).

Summary

A delayed referral for rehabilitation resulted in multiple physical and psychological complications that affected this patient's recovery. This case study clearly demonstrates the psychological implications that can result from an amputation. Most of the physiotherapy intervention was based on regaining the patient's trust in order to educate her and to provide the support that she needed to facilitate recovery. The physical exercises that were employed were relatively simple, and had they been commenced immediately after the injury, some of the complications could have been avoided.

References

Boone DC, Azen SP, Lin CM (1978) Reliability of goniometric measurements. Physical Therapy 58: 1355-60.

Boscheinen-Morrin J, Connolly WB (2001) The Hand: Fundamentals of Therapy (third edition). Oxford: Butterworth-Heinemann.

Boulas HJ (1998), Amputations of the fingers and hand: indications for replantation. Journal of the American Academy of Orthopedic Surgeons 6(2): 100-5.

Cheshire L (2000) Psychosocial aspects of hand therapy. In: M Salter, L Cheshire (eds) Hand Therapy: Principles and Practice. Oxford: Butterworth-Heinemann.

Field T, Peck M, Krugman S, Tuchel T, Schanberg S, Kuhn C et al. (1998) Burn injuries benefit from massage therapy. Journal of Burn Care and Rehabilitation 19(3): 241-4.

Jones S (1997) The prosthetist's role in partial finger loss. British Journal of Hand Therapy 2(7): 20-1.

Otthiers J (1998) Rehabilitation of ligamentous injuries of the wrist. British Journal of Hand Therapy 3(3): 6-7.

Palmada M, Shah S, O'Hare K (1999) Hand oedema: pathophysiology and treatment. British Journal of Hand Therapy 4(1): 26-32.

Parsley C (1998) The progression of reflex sympathetic dystrophy and the implications for therapy. British Journal of Hand Therapy 3(1): 14-16.

Salter M, Bexon C (2000) Treatment. In: M Salter, L Cheshire (eds) Hand Therapy: Principles and Practice. Oxford: Butterworth-Heinemann.

Small J, Brennen M, Colville J (1989) Early active mobilisation following flexor tendon repair in zone 2. Journal of Hand Surgery 14B: 383-91.

Sorenson MK (1989) The edematous hand. Physical Therapy 69(12): 1059-64.

Case study 3: Physiotherapy after burn injury

Demographic outline

A 78-year-old man was transferred to the regional burns unit, via the Accident and Emergency Department, after sustaining flash burns to his hands and face. He had been attempting to light a bonfire in his garden and had thrown petrol onto the fire, causing a sudden explosion of flames as the petrol vapours ignited. The patient had a past medical history of osteoarthritis in his knees for which he had a right total knee replacement two years before this admission; other than this, he was fit and well. He did not normally require any medication, was right-handed and was a retired bank manager who shared his enjoyment of gardening with his wife.

Assessment

Once it had been established that the patient was not suffering from any systemic effects of the burn injury, for example inhalation injury, his wounds were assessed (*see* Chapter 8). On examination, the total body surface area affected was estimated as 5% – using the 'rule of nines' method of calculating the extent of burn injuries. The burns extended over the face and anterior neck as well as over the entire dorsum of both hands, and the dorsal aspect of the wrist on the left hand. It was established that the burns were not circumferential so there was no immediate risk of ischaemia (*see* Chapter 4) from the tourniquet effect of eschar (Settle, 1996).

The depth of burn was initially assessed as mostly superficial as the wounds appeared bright red and were painful to touch (Bosworth, 1997). However, on further assessment, at 48 hours after the injury, when the erythema had resolved and the depth of the injury was clearer, there was an area over the dorsum of the left wrist that appeared to be deeper. Blisters had formed and, on application of pressure over the wound, capillary refill was delayed (*see* Chapter 8). These findings indicated a partial thickness loss of skin (Bosworth, 1997). In the centre of this area, the wound appeared white and was pain-free; this was indicative of full thickness skin loss (Bosworth, 1997).

The hands were noted to be oedematous, and circumferential measurements (*see* Chapter 8) of their size were taken as a baseline to compare with subsequent measurements. At this stage, the wounds were clean with no signs of excessive erythema, pain or odour to indicate wound infection (Kemble and Lamb, 1987).

Unlimited active range of motion was encouraged, as there was no evidence of exposed extensor tendons. The range of joint motion (see Chapter 8) achieved was initially estimated as a measurement of composite finger flexion, measuring the distance from finger pulp to palm (Boscheinen-Morrin and Conolly, 2001). However, eventually individual joint ranges were measured more accurately using goniometry. The patient's pain was assessed by use of a visual analogue scale (see Chapter 8) and his analgesic requirements were adjusted accordingly.

From the assessment of the effect of the burn injury on the patient's hands, the following priorities of intervention were established:

- pain control
- patient education
- reduction of oedema
- wound and subsequent scar management
- increase in joint range of motion
- restoration of hand function
- restoration of grip strength
- psychological support.

Goals, aims and objectives

The priority was that pain should be controlled at all times, with adequate analgesia prescribed and reviewed by the medical staff. The patient was reassured about the extent and depth of his injury and educated about the medical intervention that was needed. It was anticipated that he would gain a good level of understanding of his injury and its implications at each stage of recovery by repeated explanations and opportunities to participate in his management by questioning the team as necessary and taking an active role in decision-making and goal-setting (Downie et al., 1990).

The aim was to reduce hand oedema to a minimum and to achieve resolution by 3 months after the injury. The wounds required dressings to protect them from infection and to aid healing. Superficial areas of burn heal in 10–14 days (Bosworth, 1997); the patient's partial thickness and full thickness areas of skin loss required surgical intervention to debride and split skin graft them and these areas would heal within a week of surgery (Bosworth, 1997). The subsequent scar tissue after skin grafting should be stretched to maintain its pliability, and scar contractures over the dorsum of the wrist should be avoided (Settle, 1996).

Joint range of motion should be monitored frequently and full motion maintained at all costs. By maintaining joint motion, the patient would be able to resume hand function even while the dressings were still in place and this, in turn, would aid the maintenance of grip strength (Gairns and Martin, 1990).

The ultimate objective of rehabilitation was for the patient to return to full independence, managing his former occupation and hobbies wherever possible (Harden and Luster, 1991). To achieve this everyone, including the patient, must have a clear understanding of the aims of physiotherapy (Clarke, 1997).

Treatment

The team approach to the treatment of any hand injury is important (*see* chapters 5 and 6). Once patients' pain is controlled successfully they are able to co-operate with their treatment plans. The patient's hand oedema was reduced to prevent the complication of reduced tissue perfusion caused by raised intra-digital pressure (Trofino, 1991) and contracture. If oedema is allowed to persist, it collects in the dorsum of the hand (*see* Chapter 7). This dorsal collection would pull the hand into a clawed position, which would allow the joint structures to rest in their shortened positions and make them vulnerable to contracture (Boscheinen-Morrin et al., 1992). Contracture of these delicate structures can cause a reduction in available joint motion. By maintaining strict elevation above the level of the heart, and with active finger exercise, the oedema was reduced (*see* Chapter 9).

The burn wound was covered in silver sulphazadine and dressed in a Gore-Tex bag to prevent infection and skin maceration plus facilitate range of motion exercises, maintenance of grip strength and hand function (Gairns and Martin, 1990). The patient was able to achieve virtually the full active range of joint flexion and extension in all the joints of his hands and wrists. Therefore, it was decided that splinting the hand in a position of safe immobilization (*see* Chapter 7) was unnecessary. Allowing the patient to freely exercise the hands and use them functionally was of greater benefit (Kealey and Jensen, 1988). However, the hands needed to be monitored closely to ensure that joint motion was maintained.

Once the wounds had healed, and scar tissue had begun to develop, the patient was encouraged to continue regular active and passive exercise (*see* Chapter 9) to stretch the scar tissue (Azad et al., 2000). He was also taught to massage the scar tissue and was supplied with silicone gel and pressure garments (*see* Chapter 9) by the occupational therapist (Azad et al., 2000). In addition, the occupational therapist began to restore the patient's confidence, muscle power and hand function in the department workshop.

Throughout the whole rehabilitation process, the patient was offered emotional support by being given the opportunity to talk about his injury and the progress that was being made. Achieving the treatment goals served to motivate and encourage him. He was referred to the clinical psychologist to help him understand and cope with the psychological effects of his injury (Bosworth, 1997).

Re-assessment and modification of treatment

After removal of the immobilizing plaster of Paris 5 days after the surgical intervention of split skin grafting to the left wrist the patient was no longer able to achieve full active motion of the hand joints. Therefore, in order to prevent joint stiffness developing, a hand-resting splint was made. This positioned the wrist at 30° extension, the metacarpophalangeal joints at 70° flexion, and the interphalangeal joints in full extension with the thumb abducted (*see* Chapter 7). The splint was worn all night and during the day when the patient was not using the hand functionally or exercising. The splint was discarded once a full active range of motion was regained.

Summary

This patient's functional outcome was dependent on an integrated team approach at all stages of his recovery (Clarke, 1997). After an injury of this type it should be expected that the patient will regain full range of motion, grip strength and hand function. However, these patients need regular reviews by burns consultants and occupational therapists to monitor the development of their scar tissue.

References

Azad SM, Gerrish J, Dziewulski P (2000) Hypertrophic scars and keloids: an overview of the aetiology and management. British Journal of Hand Therapy 5(1): 16–20.

Boscheinen-Morrin J, Davey V, Connolly WB (1992) The Hand: Fundamentals of Therapy (second edition). Oxford: Butterworth-Heinemann.

Boscheinen-Morrin J, Connolly WB (2001) The Hand: Fundamentals of Therapy (third edition). Oxford: Butterworth-Heinemann.

Bosworth C (1997) Burns Trauma, Management and Nursing Care. London: Baillière Tindall.

Clarke J (1997) Burns to the hands – the perspective from Roehampton. British Journal of Hand Therapy 2(6): 9–10.

Downie RS, Fyfe C, Tannahill A (1990) Health Promotion: Models and Values. Oxford: Oxford University Press.

Gairns CE, Martin DL (1990) The use of semi-permeable membrane bags as hand burn dress-ings. Physiotherapy 76(6): 351-2.

Harden NG, Luster SH (1991) Rehabilitation considerations in the care of the acute burn patient. Critical Care Nursing Clinics of North America 3(2): 245-53.

Kealey GP, Jensen KT (1988) Aggressive approach to physical therapy management of the burned hand. Physical Therapy 68(5): 683-5.

Kemble JVH, Lamb BE (1987) Practical Burns Management. London: Hodder & Stoughton.

Settle JAD (1996) Principles and Practice of Burns Management. London: Churchill Livingstone.

Trofino RB (1991) Nursing Care of the Burn Injured Patient. Philadelphia, PA: FA Davies.

Case study 4: Physiotherapy after a groin flap

Demographic outline

A 49-year-old man sustained a degloving injury to the dorsum of his dominant right hand in machinery at work. He had no relevant past medical history and did not take any regular medication. He lived with his wife and did not have any children. After his injury he was admitted to the plastic surgery unit via the Accident and Emergency Department.

Initial examination by the medical team showed that the dorsal skin was degloved from just proximal to the wrist up to the metacarpopha-langeal joints of the fingers. The flap of degloved skin was distally based and appeared vascular as bleeding and capillary blanching was observed. The digits were also noted to be perfused and warm. The extensor digitorum tendons were exposed on the dorsum of the hand but were intact.

Initially, the degloved skin was repositioned in theatre, after debridement and irrigation to remove any contamination. The hand was then left exposed to allow close observation of the perfusion of the skin. However, over the next 2–3 days, the capillary refill rate of the skin was less than 1 second (Edwards, 1994) and the skin colour changed to a dusky blue. Venous congestion was diagnosed and leeches were used in an attempt to aid venous drainage (Valauri, 1991). Unfortunately this was unsuccessful and, on the fourth day after the accident, the patient returned to theatre for debridement of the necrotic degloved tissue and application of a groin flap to obtain wound closure. As there were exposed extensor tendons within the wound, a split skin graft was not appropriate (see Chapter 4) as this would not survive over the relatively avascular tendons (Harvey Kemble and Lamb, 1984). The pedicled groin flap remained attached to the hand for 3 weeks before it was divided and inset (McGregor and McGregor, 1995).

Assessment

The first physiotherapy assessment was made on the day after the injury when the degloved skin had been repositioned. The patient was obviously still very shocked but in good spirits probably owing to a lack of appreciation of the severity of the injury. The hand was oedematous but could not be elevated because of the risk of compromising the arterial supply to the skin. Motion of the digits was contraindicated because of the tension that this would exert on the fragile skin. The first physiotherapy assessment therefore consisted of establishing a good history from the patient and beginning to build rapport. The extent of the patient's knowledge and understanding of the severity of his injury and its implications were also ascertained from general discussion. The patient was very keen to go home and his priority was returning to work as soon as possible.

After the failure of the skin and the reconstruction of the dorsum of the hand with a groin flap, physiotherapy assessment could be more thorough, as the vasculature of the groin flap was relatively stable (McGregor and McGregor, 1995). On the first day post-operatively, the patient's respiratory state was assessed to exclude or establish any respiratory problems caused by the previous prolonged anaesthetic. He did not smoke and had no previous respiratory conditions; on examination, his chest was clear.

The position in which the hand was attached to the groin flap meant that the shoulder was positioned in slight abduction, the elbow and wrist were flexed, the metacarpophalangeal joints of the fingers were flexed and resting on the patient's hip with the palm facing upwards, whereas the interphalangeal joints of the fingers were in a slightly flexed position. The thumb was also in a relaxed position. Range of motion exercises at the shoulder, elbow and wrist were minimal because of the risk of creating tension on the pedicle of the groin flap. Extension of the metacarpophalangeal joints of the fingers was prevented by their position resting on the patient's hip. Active motion of the interphalangeal joints of the digits and the three joints of the thumb was possible, but objective measurement with goniometry was impractical owing to the position of the hand. Therefore, estimated measurements of the distance between the fingertips and distal palmar crease of the hand were made (Boscheinen-Morrin and Connolly, 2001). Full passive motion of the thumb and interphalangeal joints of the fingers was possible, but the patient required a lot of reassurance and explanation before this was attempted. The hand remained oedematous but again, it was impractical to attempt any objective measurement of the swelling.

Priorities

From the assessment, the priorities for the physiotherapeutic care of this patient were:

- education, reassurance and encouragement
- oedema control
- positioning to avoid tension or kinking of the flap
- maintenance of range of motion of digits and joints of the upper limb
- gait re-education
- restoration of function.

Goals, aims and objectives

The most important objective of the multidisciplinary team was that the patient would understand the treatment programme and not only comply but also take an active role in the decision-making processes (Ashe, 2001). The first priority was that the groin flap should not be compromised by any therapeutic intervention so the treatment programme was designed around maintenance of the flap.

Physiotherapy intervention aimed to maintain as much of the range of motion in all of the joints of the upper limb as was possible (Ranelli et al., 2000). Because of the position of immobilization during the 3 weeks before flap division, range of motion was limited in all but the interphalangeal joints of the fingers and the whole of the thumb. The goal of treatment during this time was to achieve full range of motion in the joints that were free to move. It was felt that even though there was not any tendon damage there was the potential for the tendons to become tethered in interstructural adhesions (Small et al., 1989). By moving the free joints of the fingers, the tendons would glide and therefore prevent this tethering (Ranelli, 1998). Once the flap was divided, the aim of treatment was to restore as much range of motion in the other joints as was possible.

As oedema could not be restricted by elevation until flap division (McGregor and McGregor, 1995), the aim of the treatment programme was to minimize its development and to limit its adverse effects (Palmada et al., 1999). After flap division the emphasis of rehabilitation became more functional in order to restore the patient's ability to perform activities of daily living. Functional goal-setting was used to aid motivation (Salter and Cheshire, 2000).

Treatment programme

The medical team and specialist plastic surgery nurses gave a full explanation of the care of the flap to the patient. This was reiterated by the physiotherapist, and the patient was given time to ask questions and voice any concerns about his treatment. The main concern that was expressed by the patient was that he would have to remain in hospital for 3 weeks before the flap was divided. It was explained to the patient that the flap would be closely observed for the next 2–3 days and that after that if it remained satisfactory and if he had achieved the agreed goals with the physiotherapist he would be able to go home and attend the outpatient dressing and physiotherapy clinics.

To achieve the goals the patient commenced his treatment programme on the first day after surgery. In order to reduce hand oedema and maintain joint range of motion, active and passive movements were commenced (Palmada et al., 1999). These included shoulder girdle movements, such as elevation, protraction, retraction and circumduction. Minimal elbow joint motion was available owing to the position of the limb, but a degree of wrist flexion and extension was possible if the hand was supported. Active and gentle passive finger interphalangeal joint motion was initiated, as was thumb motion, however, finger metacarpophalangeal joint motion was restricted because of the position of the hand and concern about placing too much tension on the flap.

At 48 hours after surgery, the patient was allowed to start mobilizing. The arm was secured with strapping to prevent any tension on the pedicle as he stood, and he was advised to maintain a slightly flexed posture rather than standing up straight. Initially, the patient felt a little dizzy because of his enforced bed rest for the last few days. This passed after he was allowed to sit upright for a few minutes and when he began to walk, he did not require any assistance. The patient was discharged home 4 days after surgery. He then attended the dressing and physiotherapy clinics every other day to check his progress.

Re-assessment and alterations to treatment programme

Three weeks after surgery the patient returned to theatre to have the groin flap divided and partially inset (McGregor and McGregor, 1995). On the day after surgery, the dressings were removed and the upper limb could be examined. On assessment, the patient did not have any pain. The range of shoulder motion was limited into lateral rotation, flexion and abduction. There was full range of motion at the elbow joint although the patient did complain of some stiffness. Wrist extension was limited to neutral, thumb range of motion was full and finger motion was full at the interphalangeal joints but metacarpophalangeal joint extension was poor. Range of motion was assessed using goniometry (Boone et al., 1978). The hand was oedematous but volumetric measurements as described by Boland and Adams (1996) were not deemed appropriate because of the open wounds and because any atrophy of the flap would distort subsequent volumetric measurements. It was decided that circumferential measurement would give a more accurate indication of oedema resolution in the digits, and these measurements were compared with the contralateral hand (*see* Chapter 8). Wound assessment demonstrated a healthy granulating edge to the flap where some of its periphery had not been inset to avoid placing tension on the vasculature (McGregor and McGregor, 1995). This was covered with a light; non-adherent gauze dressing that did not restrict joint motion.

Despite the presence of oedema, a light compression dressing (Coban) was only applied to the digits. Compression was contraindicated over the flap because of its possible effect on flap perfusion (Edwards, 1994). At 5 weeks after reconstructive surgery, the flap was deemed stable and a compression glove was used to aid drainage of the residual oedema (Palmada et al., 1999).

Active shoulder, elbow, wrist and hand exercise was commenced on the day after flap division. The patient was encouraged to exercise hourly, and was taught to use auto-assisted techniques to achieve full shoulder range of motion. Gentle passive wrist and metacarpophalangeal joint extension was included in the treatment programme, as this did not create any tension in the flap. The different grip postures of full, hook, flat and straight fist (*see* Chapter 9) were used to achieve differential tendon gliding (Sorenson, 1989). Active metacarpophalangeal joint extension with interphalangeal joint flexion was used in an attempt to gain glide of the extensor digitorum tendons beneath the flap (Ranelli, 1998). Abduction and adduction of the fingers was used also to maintain tendon gliding but mainly to reduce oedema by utilizing the hand muscle pumps (Simons et al., 1996). Light functional activities were encouraged immediately and the patient was referred to the occupational therapy department to facilitate this (McGourty et al., 1986).

The main difficulty experienced by the patient was regaining wrist extension. On assessment, this was found to be due to carpal and radio-carpal stiffness rather than to soft tissue tethering, as wrist range of motion was limited despite the position of the finger joints. This was probably because of the prolonged immobility of the wrist in a flexed position during the inflammatory and proliferative phase of healing. Carpal and radio-carpal mobilizations (*see* Chapter 9) were used in order to release some of this joint stiffness (Maitland, 1992) and were found to be effective.

Strengthening exercises for the hand were commenced and gradually upgraded from the first week after the division of the flap. However, the patient found that functional use of the hand facilitated the restoration of his grip strength rather than specific exercise.

Once the flap had healed, the patient was instructed in scar tissue massage (Ronon, 2001) for the edges of the flap and the donor site scar. The patient found this easier to incorporate into his regular exercise programme with the gentle retrograde massage that he was using for oedema dispersal (Sorenson, 1989). He did not require silicone gel.

By 8 weeks after the injury, the patient had achieved full pain-free shoulder and elbow joint range of motion. At the wrist, he had full flexion and 50° extension. Full range of motion had been maintained in the thumb and the interphalangeal joints of the fingers but metacarpophalangeal joint extension was still limited to neutral in the index and middle fingers and lacked 10° and 15° in the ring and little fingers, respectively. He returned to work on light duties and was discharged from physiotherapy but advised to continue his exercise programme and his attendance at occupational therapy.

Summary

This challenging case required the physiotherapist to re-think the tried and tested ways of treating major hand trauma, that is, elevation and early active motion. The limitations of the situation meant that therapy needed to be monitored carefully to ensure that it did not put the skin flap at risk of failure but prevented the consequences of immobility. By assessing and reassessing the treatment options, plus altering the treatment plan as the surgical intervention progressed, the physiotherapist was able to achieve the aim of restoring upper limb range of motion and function. By involvement with the patient from the admission through the in- and outpatient treatment phases, the physiotherapist was in a position to support the patient not only with his rehabilitation needs but also his psychological adjustment.

A team approach to the care of this patient was essential at every stage of his treatment and this was facilitated with regular multidisciplinary meetings to maintain communication between the team members. The physiotherapists required information from the medical and nursing staff relating to the state of the flap so that the vascular supply was not compromised with treatment. The occupational therapist and physiotherapist needed to work closely together to ensure that the information that they gave to the patient was consistent, and that their treatments complemented each other. Referral to the clinical psychologist was essential to enable the patient to express his emotions and learn to overcome his injury.

Even after this devastating injury and complicated reconstruction, it was expected that the patient would regain enough joint motion and strength to resume his pre-injury activities. His determination was such that he achieved an adequate range of motion in his upper limb joints to return to work on light duties whilst still attending occupational therapy to regain the strength that was required for full function.

References

Ashe MC (2001) Management of carpal instability: a therapist's perspective. British Journal of Hand Therapy 6(1): 9-14.

Boland R, Adams R (1996) Development and evaluation of a precision forearm and hand volumeter and measuring cylinder. Journal of Hand Therapy 9(4): 349-58.

Boone DC, Azen SP, Lin CM (1978) Reliability of goniometric measurements. Physical Therapy 58: 1355-60.

Boscheinen-Morrin J, Connolly WB (2001) The Hand: Fundamentals of Therapy (third edition). Oxford: Butterworth-Heinemann.

Edwards K (1994) Skin flaps in plastic surgery: an overview. Nursing Standard 9(4): 27-30.

Harvey Kemble JV, Lamb BE (1984) Plastic Surgical and Burns Nursing. London: Baillière Tindall.

Maitland G (1992) Peripheral Manipulation (eighth edition). Edinburgh: Churchill Livingstone.

McGourty LK, Givens A, Fader PB (1986) Roles and functions of occupational therapy in burn care delivery. Journal of Burn Care and Rehabilitation 7(5): 431-3.

McGregor IA, McGregor AD (1995) Fundamental Techniques of Plastic Surgery and their Surgical Applications. Edinburgh: Churchill Livingstone.

Palmada M, Shah S, O'Hare K (1999) Hand oedema: pathophysiology and treatment. British Journal of Hand Therapy 4(1): 26-32.

Ranelli S (1998) Controlled active extension programme in association with dynamic splinting for extensor tendon reconstruction zones three-eight. British Journal of Hand Therapy 3(1): 12-13.

Ranelli S, Forsythe S, Nanchahal J (2000) Principles of rehabilitation in reconstructive surgery in the upper limb. British Journal of Hand Therapy 5(1): 5-9.

Ronon C (2001) The use of massage to influence collagen synthesis in the hand: a physiological justification. British Journal of Hand Therapy 6(3): 95-9.

Salter M, Cheshire L (2000) Hand Therapy, Principles and Practice. Oxford: Butterworth-Heinemann.

Simons P, Coleridge Smith P, Lees WR, McGrowther DA (1996) Venous pumps of the hand: their clinical importance. Journal of Hand Surgery 21B: 595-9.

Small J, Brennen M, Colville J (1989) Early active mobilisation following flexor tendon repair in zone 2. Journal of Hand Surgery 14B: 383-91.

Sorenson MK (1989) The edematous hand. Physical Therapy 69(12): 1054-64.

Valauri FA (1991) The use of medicinal leeches in microsurgery. Blood Coagulation and Fibrinolysis 2: 185-7.

Case study 5: Physiotherapy after replantation

Demographic outline

A 50-year-old left-handed male manual worker sustained a traumatic amputation of his left hand with a circular saw at mid-shaft level of the metacarpal bones. The ulnar three digits were replanted four and a half hours after the injury. The patient was fit and well before his accident. He had no relevant past medical history or associated injuries that might have precluded prolonged microvascular surgery (Lister, 1992). The amputated hand had been transported to the hospital and then stored in the ideal way. It was wrapped in sterile gauze, placed in a clean plastic bag and then placed into another plastic bag with cold water and ice (Strauch et al., 1986). Care had been taken to avoid direct contact with the ice to prevent frostbite and cold damage to the tissues. There had been no extreme contamination, lengthy warm ischaemia or previous injury or surgery to the amputated part. The injury was a 'clean cut' and there was no extensive vascular damage to either the affected limb or the amputated part that would contra-indicate replantation (Wilson, 1983). Results obtained from replantation were therefore expected to be worth the investment in replantation surgery and rehabilitation (Wilson, 1983).

Following the pre-operative assessment and preparation, two surgeons simultaneously identified and labelled the structures of the amputated part and the stump. The patient's thumb was uninjured but there was such gross destruction of the second metacarpophalangeal joint that his index finger was discarded. In a 10.5-hour operation, the surgeons shortened the second metacarpal as for a Ray amputation, and fixed the third, fourth and fifth metacarpals with interosseous wires and oblique K-wires to establish a solid base. They then repaired the common digital arteries to the third and fourth web spaces, made four venous anastomoses, sutured the long flexor and extensor tendons, repaired all of the digital nerves and finally closed the skin.

Assessment

Post-operatively, the hand was nursed horizontally to prevent any decrease in arterial blood flow. Plastic surgery nurses checked frequently for signs of inadequate circulation (Coull and Wylie, 1990) in order to take prompt action to prevent failure of the replant if necessary (*see* Chapter 4).

Physiotherapy assessment of the affected limb took place on the first day after surgery. Range of motion of the elbow and shoulder was assessed using goniometry (Boone et al., 1978) and was found to be full. The hand was placed in a splint in a position of safe immobilization (*see* Chapter 7) in order to prevent damage of the repaired structures but with care not to exert pressure on the vascular anastamoses (Ranelli et al., 2000). Motion of the hand was not commenced until the fifth day postoperatively; goniometry was used to evaluate range. It was impractical to measure hand oedema with a volumeter (Boland and Adams, 1996) because of the delicate state of the tissues, therefore circumferential measurements were taken (*see* Chapter 8) and compared with measurements from the contralateral hand.

It was inappropriate to assess muscle strength and function at this early stage of the patient's recovery. Once the patient was able to commence strengthening exercises (at 10–12 weeks) the Jamar dynamometer was used to monitor his recovery (*see* Chapter 8). To assess the patient's functional recovery the Disabilities of the Arm, Shoulder and Hand (DASH) questionnaire was used (Hudak et al., 1996). This was chosen because it was quick to use and reflected the patient's perception of his functional ability rather than the physiotherapist's interpretation (*see* Chapter 8).

Problems identified and priorities

From the initial assessment, the aims of physiotherapy were noted to be:

- prevention of post-operative respiratory complications
- maintenance of range of motion at the elbow and shoulder joints
- prevention of joint stiffness in the wrist and hand
- prevention of soft tissue adhesions and maintenance of tendon glide
- restoration of as full function as possible
- provision of psychological support.

Goals, aims and objectives

The initial aim of physiotherapy was to protect the hand in order to promote survival of the replanted parts. Recent published literature documents the survival rate of replanted parts of the upper limb as between 80% (Doyle et al., 1989) and 90% (Weinzweig et al., 1996) with a greater survival rate for clean-cut wounds with less than 12 hours' ischaemic time (Razana et al., 1998). Although the results of replantation surgery were once judged upon cosmesis, emphasis is now placed on functional outcome. Chow et al. (1983) stated that functional recovery after replantation is dependent on two factors: the degree of nerve degeneration and the hand rehabilitation programme. In a small Mexican study, satisfactory functional recovery was achieved in only 50% of cases (Romero-Zarate et al., 2000). However, if patients are selected appropriately for replantation surgery the results achieved should be better than current prosthetic devises (Doyle et al., 1989).

This patient's ultimate goal was to be able to return to his previous employment as soon as possible. In order to achieve this he needed to understand his limitations and accept the slow progression of treatment. Full range of motion at the elbow and shoulder joints was achieved on the first day after surgery but this motion needed to be maintained throughout his treatment. Some joint stiffness and loss of tendon glide in the hand and wrist was inevitable (Lister, 1992). However, the treatment aim was to maintain as much range of motion as was necessary for the patient to resume functional activity.

Maintaining the patient's mental health was a priority. In order to prevent and treat any psychological problems the clinical psychologist was involved in the patient's care immediately.

Treatment programme

Because of the lengthy anaesthesia, and because the patient smoked 20 cigarettes a day, the first post-operative day physiotherapy sessions were focused on respiratory assessment and chest clearance techniques. The patient was advised to stop smoking, not only for his respiratory welfare but also to avoid the risks of thrombosis and delayed healing (Reus et al., 1992) as nicotine is also known to be a vasoconstrictor (Van Adrichem et al., 1992).

For the first four post-operative days, the patient maintained shoulder and elbow joint range of movement with regular active exercise. He also wore a hand-resting splint to prevent any tension on the repaired structures and to prevent the joint structures from contracting (Kennedy et al., 1998). The wrist was positioned in neutral, the metacarpophalangeal joints at 40°, and the interphalangeal joints in extension.

The development of extensive oedema was exacerbated by the requirement of the horizontal positioning of the limb. Ideally, active and passive movements should be started as soon as possible to aid dispersion of oedema (Nicholas, 1977; Palmada et al., 1999), prevent joint stiffness, limit soft tissue adhesions and maintain tendon glide (Cullen et al., 1989). However, movement was not commenced until the fifth post-operative day because of the risk of disrupting the arterial anastomoses (Burke, 1983).

After discussion with the surgeons, an exercise programme was devised:

- four protected passive flexions of metacarpophalangeal joints
- four protected passive flexions of the interphalangeal joints
- two active combined flexions of all digits together.

This set of exercises was performed four times a day. Between exercise sessions, the hand-resting splint was replaced. Once the risks of compromising the circulation had passed, oedema was controlled with elasticated bandages (Simons et al., 1996) and gentle retrograde massage (Sorenson, 1989). This treatment programme was followed until the patient was discharged home 10 days after surgery.

The patient had a good understanding of his exercise programme and was motivated. Full protected passive flexion and extension of the interphalangeal joints could be achieved and approximately three-quarters range of protected passive flexion and extension at the metacarpophalangeal joints. Active movement was also improving. The patient was instructed to perform the exercise programme four times a day, was warned of the risks associated with anaesthetic skin and the risk of tendon rupture, and was taught skin care. He attended physiotherapy as an outpatient daily and progressed satisfactorily.

Three weeks after the operation, combined metacarpophalangeal and interphalangeal joint active and gentle passive flexion and extension of the digits was included in the exercise programme, which was increased to hourly sessions as the tendons were deemed strong enough to withstand this stress (Strickland, 1989). The resting splint was also removed during the day to allow active wrist exercise and light functional activities. A functional bias was incorporated into the exercise programme and occupational therapy offered further assistance with functional exercises. Oedema was a persistent problem and a pressure garment was fitted to control this (Kennedy et al., 2000).

The K-wires were removed 6 weeks after replantation. As the patient was attending the occupational therapy workshop regularly, it was decided to reduce his attendance at the physiotherapy department to twice a week. Maintenance of wrist extension continued to be a problem during gripping activities; therefore, a splint to support his wrist in slight extension was supplied (Duncan, 1989).

Twelve weeks is generally accepted as the point at which the tendons are healed and the treatment programme was progressed to incorporate resisted exercises to regain lost grip strength (Peck et al., 1998). The proximal interphalangeal joints were beginning to contract into flexion, but as this flexed position was considered more functional than full extension, they were monitored but not corrected.

The patient was discharged from physiotherapy 16 weeks after his replantation. Heavy objects presented his only functional difficulty but this and his strength was continuing to improve with occupational therapy. He had returned to work on a part-time basis.

Progress report and alterations to regime

Initially, rehabilitation was limited by the need for protected motion because of the delicate tendon repairs (Cullen et al., 1989). For example, while actively or passively flexing the joints, consideration was given to the extensor tendon repairs, which would be stretched during this manoeuvre. Hence, any passive movements had to be in a protected position to prevent overstretch and rupture of repaired tendons, for example during passive flexion of the interphalangeal joints, the metacarpophalangeal joints and wrist were positioned in extension to reduce the tension on the extensor tendons. The patient was gradually encouraged to take responsibility for his own exercises under the supervision of physiotherapist.

Although the patient had lost digital sensibility, motor control was undamaged because of the site of the injury. If the injury had been more proximal, that is, at or proximal to the wrist, not only would the amputated part have been more vulnerable to ischaemic damage but the rehabilitation programme would also have required passive movements to maintain range of movement, which could not be achieved actively because of the denervation of muscles. A longer rehabilitation programme would have been necessary to re-educate the muscles as they became re-innervated with nerve growth.

It was unusual in this case that the patient never reported any symptoms of post-traumatic stress disorder. Signs indicating psychological distress, such as flashbacks of the accident, anxiety and grief, have been demonstrated as early as on admission to the Accident and Emergency Department (Grunert et al., 1992). Although it is not within the realm of physiotherapists to provide counselling, in order for them to make an appropriate referral to other professionals it is necessary that they should be able to recognize the signs of psychological distress (*see* Chapter 9).

The consultant discharged this patient from the clinic 2 years after his injury. He had no functional deficit and had returned to his previous employment. This compares favourably to Weinzweig et al. (1996), who noted that none of the 13 trans-metacarpal replantations in their study was able to return to manual labour. The patient's range of movement remained limited yet adequate and he had full muscle power. Protective sensation had returned to the tips of his digits. This patient's attitude and motivation were such that he achieved an excellent result after a potentially devastating injury. He now helps to counsel patients who have suffered similar injuries.

It must always be kept in mind that when assessing the outcome of a replanted hand, it should not be compared with the uninjured hand but with the only other option available to the surgeon, that of terminalization of the stump. However, when the outcome of the patient in this case study was compared to Lister's (1992) expectations, it was clear that he achieved an above-average result. Lister (1992) stated that, on average, a patient required 7 months off work, that the motion in the joints of the replanted part would average 50% of normal and that some 60% of patients required an average of 2.5 further operations.

Summary

There is a lack of a widely accepted rehabilitation protocol for patients after replantation surgery and therefore the treatment of individual patients must be based on knowledge of average healing times of damaged structures, risk factors and safe practice. The rehabilitation programme should be individual for particular patients and injury (Silverman and Gordon, 1996). The progression of treatment for one of the damaged structures may be contraindicated because of the risk it would place on another of the structures. Factors that need to be considered are the nature of the injury, the structures repaired, the state of the tissues and the differing healing times of the tissues. Physiotherapists need to combine all of their anatomical, pathological and biomechanical knowledge with their skills in problem-solving to facilitate the best possible outcome for these patients. A team approach to the care of this patient was essential. The surgeons were able to give information on the state of the repaired tissues, the nurses dressed and monitored the hand for signs of failure, the dietician ensured the patient received the nutrition required for tissue repair, the physiotherapist and occupational therapist guided the rehabilitation and the psychologist maintained the patient's mental health. However, the patient managed to come to terms with his injury and maintain motivation to follow his treatment programme.

References

Boland R, Adams R (1996) Development and evaluation of a precision forearm and hand volumeter and measuring cylinder. Journal of Hand Therapy 9(4): 349–58.
Burke FD (1983) Microsurgery in the upper limb. Physiotherapy 69(10): 3469.
Chow JA, Bilos LJ, Chunpiapaph B, Hui P (1983) Forearm replantation: long-term functional results. Annals of Plastic Surgery 10: 15.

Coull A, Wylie K (1990) Regular monitoring: the way to ensure flap healing, nursing priorities following flap repair and reconstruction surgery. Professional Nurse October: 18–21.

Cullen KW, Tolhurst P, Lang D, Page RE (1989) Flexor tendon repair in zone 2 by controlled active mobilisation. Journal of Hand Surgery 14B: 392–5.

Doyle JR, Seitz WH, McBride M (1989) Replantation. Hand Clinics 5(3): 415–21.

Duncan RM (1989) Basic principles of splinting the hand. Physical Therapy 69(11): 1104–16.

Grunert BK, Devine CA, Smith CJ, Matloub HS, Sanger JR, Yousif NJ (1992) Graded work exposure to promote work return after severe hand trauma: a replicated study. Annals of Plastic Surgery 29(6): 532–6.

Hudak PL, Amadio PC, Bombardier C (1996) Development of an upper extremity outcome measure: the DASH (disabilities of the arm, shoulder and hand). American Journal of Industrial Medicine 29: 602–8.

Kennedy S, Peck F, Stone J (1998) Prophylactic splintage of the 5th metacarpophalangeal joint in dorsal hand burns. British Journal of Hand Therapy 3(4): 22–3.

Kennedy S, Peck F, Stone J (2000) The treatment of interphalangeal joint flexion contractures with reinforced lycra finger sleeves. British Journal of Hand Therapy 5(2): 46–8.

Lister G (1992) The Hand: Diagnosis and Indications (third edition). Edinburgh: Churchill Livingstone.

Nicholas JS (1977) The swollen hand. Physiotherapy 63(9): 285–6.

Palmada M, Shah S, O'Hare K (1999) Hand oedema: pathophysiology and treatment. British Journal of Hand Therapy 4(1): 26–32.

Peck FH, Bucher CA, Watson JS, Roe A (1998) A comparative study of two methods of controlled mobilisation of flexor tendon repairs in zone 2. Journal of Hand Surgery 23B(1): 41–5.

Ranelli S, Forsythe S, Nanchahal J (2000) Principles of rehabilitation in reconstructive surgery in the upper limb. British Journal of Hand Therapy 5(1): 5–9.

Razana A, Hyzan MY, Pathmanathan V, Gill RS (1998) Hand replantation and revascularisation – six years experience in Hospital Kuala Lumpur 1990–1995. Medical Journal of Malaysia 53 (Suppl. A): 121–30.

Reus WF, Colen LB, Straker DJ (1992) Tobacco smoking and complications in elective microsurgery. Plastic and Reconstructive Surgery 89(3): 490–4.

Romero-Zarate JL, Pastrana-Figueroa JM, Granados-Martinez R (2000) Upper extremity replantation: three year experience. Microsurgery 20(4): 202–6.

Silverman PM, Gordon L (1996) Early motion after replantation. Hand Clinics 12(1): 97–107.

Simons P, Coleridge Smith P, Lees WR, McGrowther DA (1996) Venous pumps of the hand: their clinical importance. Journal of Hand Surgery 21B: 595–9.

Sorenson MK (1989) The edematous hand. Physical Therapy 69(12): 1059–64.

Strauch B, Greinstein B, Goldstein R, Liebling RW (1986) Problems and complications encountered in replantation surgery. Hand Clinics 2(2): 389–99.

Strickland JW (1989) Biologic rationale, clinical application, and results of early motion following flexor tendon repair. Journal of Hand Therapy Apr–Jun: 71–83.

Tittle BJ, English JM, Hodges PL (1993) Microsurgery: free tissue transfer and replantation. Selected Readings in Plastic Surgery 7(11): 14–21.

Van Adrichem LNA, Hovius SER, van Strik R, van der Muelen JC (1992) The effect of cigarette smoking on the microcirculation of a replanted digit. Journal of Hand Surgery 17A(2): 230–3.

Wilson CS (1983) Replantation of the upper extremity. Clinics in Plastic Surgery 10: 85–101.

Weinzweig N, Sharzer LA, Starker I (1996) Replantation and revascularisation at the trans-metacarpal level: long-term functional results. Journal of Hand Surgery 21A(5): 877–83.

Appendix

Useful addresses

- Burn Survivor Association (www.burnsurvivorassociation.com)
- Chartered Society of Physiotherapy, 14 Bedford Row, London WC1R 4ED
- College of Occupational Therapists, 106–114 Borough High Street, Southwark, London SE1 1LB
- British Burns Association, Mrs S Hodgkinson, PO Box 74, Morpeth, Northumberland NE65 8YT
- British Association of Hand Therapists, 923 Finchley Road, London NW11 7PE
- British Association of Plastic Surgeons, The Royal College of Surgeons, Lincoln's Inn Fields, London WC2A 3PN

Index